A PLUME BOOK

PART-TIME PALEO

LEANNE ELY, CNC, is the founder of SavingDinner.com, the original menu-planning website that's been online since 2001. She is a national spokesperson for Meals on Wheels and the founder of the Take Back the Dinner Table movement. She lives in Charlotte, North Carolina.

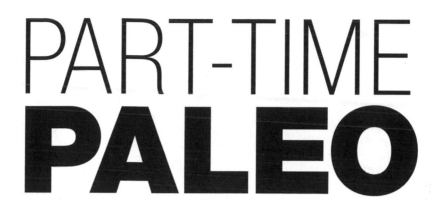

PART-TIME
PALEO

HOW TO GO PALEO
WITHOUT GOING CRAZY

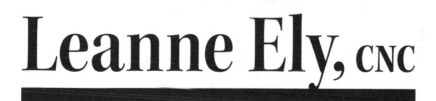

Leanne Ely, CNC

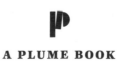

A PLUME BOOK

PLUME
Published by the Penguin Group
Penguin Group (USA) LLC
375 Hudson Street
New York, New York 10014

USA | Canada | UK | Ireland | Australia | New Zealand | India | South Africa | China
penguin.com
A Penguin Random House Company

First published by Plume, a member of Penguin Group (USA) LLC, 2014

P REGISTERED TRADEMARK—MARCA REGISTRADA

ISBN 978-0-14-218066-2

Printed in the United States of America
10   9   8   7   6   5   4   3   2   1

Set in Kepler Std with Helvetica Neue LT Std
Designed by Daniel Lagin

This book is dedicated to my mom. I'm proud to be your daughter.

CONTENTS

ACKNOWLEDGMENTS

There are many thank-yous to be given here, and I know I will invariably forget someone (please forgive me!).

First off, thank you to my amazing staff—Daniel, Sally, Angela, Cara, and the entire menu-writing team.

And of course, thank you to Jaime, whose editing and writing keeps the machine rolling!

Thank you to Jenae, my fabulous assistant, for always being on top of everything!

A special thank-you to my coach, Cameron Herold, who pushes me hard to be my best.

And to my friends and family who lived with my squirreliness throughout yet another book—thanks for putting up with me!

And lastly to my children, Caroline and Peter, and my new son-in-law, Samuel. You inspire me daily and I love you with all my heart.

INTRODUCTION

WHAT IS THE PALEO DIET?

What the heck is this Paleo diet about, anyway? Do you eat nothing but mastodon steaks grilled over an open flame?

I'm a part-time Paleoista myself, so I get asked questions like this all the time. (For the record, there are no mastodon steaks involved in the Paleo diet. But if you find a good source of local, free-range mastodon, let me know. I'll try anything once!)

The first thing you must understand is that the word *Paleo* is an abbreviated term referring to the Paleolithic age (but I bet you already knew that). This is the period in history when our ancestors ate what they could hunt, fish, or gather. That is the basis for this diet: meat, fish, eggs, and lots of veggies, berries, and nuts.

MY PERSONAL PALEO JOURNEY

Ten years ago I was diagnosed with Hashimoto's thyroiditis, an auto-immune disease that makes you feel depressed, exhausted, and generally miserable. And on top of those less-than-pleasant symptoms, Hashimoto's causes weight gain. I also have a skin condition called rosacea, which only added to my anguish, making me a cranky, overweight, depressed monster with a red face and pimples. Delightful, no?

I was stuck. I was in a vortex that was sucking me down. Everything was a struggle, and I just couldn't snap out of my sad, sorry state of mind.

As I researched autoimmune diseases, I kept reading over and over again about the Paleo diet and how it was reducing inflammation and healing people who were suffering from all sorts of autoimmune disorders, all the while helping people to lose weight and feel amazing.

When I first heard about the premise of the Paleo diet, to say I was skeptical is an understatement.

I kept thinking, "Oh, come on! I don't want to give up bread and beans and potatoes! I've already done the low-carb thing—how is this any different?"

But after reading so many success stories, I couldn't help but think that there was a chance that changing my diet would help me, just like it was helping so many other people. I shifted my thinking, and I gave myself a pep talk: "Leanne, stop thinking about what you have to give up, and start thinking about what you have to gain."

I threw myself into the Paleo diet. At first it was difficult. I missed bread, rice, and the occasional baked potato. But guess what? Things were starting to change. I started feeling better. I was feeling so good that I wanted to exercise more, which, of course, made me feel even better. I added green juicing to the mix, and I began to feel like a brand-new person.

The inflammation in my body was starting to subside and all of my symptoms were disappearing one by one. After just ten days, my skin was clearing up, I was losing weight, and my blood work was coming back with no areas of concern—and let me tell you, blood work doesn't lie.

It's been about eight years since I last wrote a book. Before that, I was writing all the time, keeping my publisher very happy. Nothing has really inspired me to write again like the Paleo diet has. And that's why you're reading this very passage. I was so inspired by my own journey that I wanted to share it with you. This is a lifestyle that really, really works.

Now, if you've been doing any amount of digging into this way of eating and living, no doubt you've come across some pretty hard-core Paleo folks (more on them in Chapter Two). If the idea of eating like this seems too stringent, just relax. There's a reason I called this book *Part-Time Paleo*!

I knew this book had to be about incorporating the best parts of the Paleo diet into your lifestyle so that it could be effective and manageable. Because let's be realistic—we can only do what we can do.

Now that you know that you don't have to live and die by a strict set of caveman rules, let's look a little deeper into the science of Paleo.

THE RESEARCH

Research has shown that our hunter-gatherer ancestors were lean, strong, and athletic and that they were afflicted with none of our modern-day maladies, such as diabetes and cancer. Interesting, yes?

Here we are in modern-day North America with our fancy medicine and billions of dollars spent on health care and research, and we are sick. Everyone knows someone with diabetes, cancer, high blood pressure, or heart disease because the Standard American Diet (SAD) is actually substandard. We are not eating enough of the right things (organic produce and grass-fed meats), and we're eating too much of the wrong things (refined sugar and processed foods).

The physiological signs that we were meant to eat Paleo are right under our noses, literally. Let's start by looking at our teeth. Our teeth tell us what we should eat. We have a combination of sharp teeth like those of carnivores and flat teeth like those of herbivores. With teeth suitable for both meat and vegetables, it's clear that we're omnivores. Lucky us! Omnivores have endless options in the food chain—we can eat meat, fish, veggies, eggs, nuts, and plants because we are naturally equipped to handle these foods. And this omnivorous diet is the wisest and best eating option for humans.

Doctors and nutritionists have been researching how eating Paleo can give us lean, healthy bodies and even reverse disease. There is evidence that a lifestyle based on a Paleo diet is beneficial on a variety of levels.

In my own research, I have found that things like legumes, grains, and processed foods, which were brought to us with the advent of agriculture, aren't as natural as we've been led to believe. These types of foods are actually hard on our bodies and can lead to chronic illness.

Since the agricultural revolution, we have drastically changed our diet to one that is very different from what is natural to our bodies. In his national best seller, *Why We Get Fat*, Gary Taubes explains, "The modern foods that today constitute more than 60 percent of all calories in the typical Western diet—including cereal grains, dairy products, beverages, vegetable oils and dressings, and sugar and candy—would have contributed virtually none of the energy in the typical hunter-gatherer diet." This change in diet, Taubes theorizes, may have made us more susceptible to a variety of diseases and dangerous health conditions. Taubes goes on to state that "colon cancer is 10 times more common in rural Connecticut than in Nigeria. Alzheimer's disease is far more common among Japanese Americans than among Japanese living in Japan."

The implication is that there is a strong connection between particular diseases and the Western diet—a diet that is very different from the one of our ancient ancestors.

Our Western way of eating is harming us. Our physiology has hardly changed in the past ten thousand years. We digest food the same way our ancestors did. But the "foods" we're putting into our bodies don't resemble the foods eaten in Paleolithic times. And it's this introduction of unrecognizable foods into our bodies that is causing harm. Our cells don't know what to do with all of the chemicals in foods like margarine and microwave popcorn.

The Paleolithic era is where we first find evidence of stone tools being used—not tools that made things more convenient, but tools they needed so they could eat, period. These tools made it easier to hunt bigger game. Eventually, we became hunter-gatherers who ate mostly meat. Researchers hypothesize that the Paleolithic age is when our genes were shaped. If our most natural state of being comes from this time period, then why don't we live accordingly?

One of the more interesting things I came across during my research is a study that was done in the 1980s called the Kitava Study. Created by Staffan Lindeberg, MD, PhD, associate professor in the Department of Medicine at Lund University, in Sweden, this study closely monitored the dietary habits of a particular Papua New Guinea tribe (the Kitava tribe). The diet of the Kitava people matched that of our Paleolithic ancestors. What the researchers found over a series of years is remarkable: "Despite a fair number of older residents, none of whom showed signs of dementia or poor memory, the only cases of sudden death the residents could recall were accidents such as drowning or falling from a coconut tree."* They did not find any accounts of heart disease, nor were there any signs of diabetes, dementia, acne, high blood pressure, strokes, or weight problems!

WHAT DO I ACTUALLY *EAT*?

So, are you ready to go Paleo and start reaping the benefits? Good. Now, let's get down to basics.

The basis of the diet is the consumption of anything our hunter-gatherer ancestors might have eaten: meat, fish, eggs, veggies, some

---

* "The Kitava Study," Paleolithic Diet In Medical Nutrition, www.staffanlindeberg.com/TheKitavaStudy .html.

fruits, and nuts and seeds. Paleoistas live without dairy, grains, and most legumes. So, you can have steak, but skip the dinner roll. You might be surprised that foods you thought were healthy, like peanuts, chickpeas, and whole grains, are forbidden by Paleoistas, but foods like beef, butter, and wine are A-OK!

When you get to the meals and recipes in this book, you'll see that we Paleoistas use delicious methods of cooking and add herbs and spices to our food. We enjoy liberal use of olive and coconut oils, balsamic vinegar, and some assorted condiments when appropriate (like Dijon mustard or salsa, for example). Paleo eating is naturally gluten-free and low glycemic. Eggs appear frequently in the diet, as does nitrate/nitrite-free bacon. Did I just hear an amen?

Before you start to panic about what you can and cannot eat, relax! As you adjust to this new way of living (yes, this is a lifestyle and not a diet), I'm going to help you as much as I can. Remember, once upon a time I was in the exact mental place as you are now.

PART-TIME PALEO RULES

Here are the basic rules you will follow as a Part-Time Paleo eater:

1. **Skip the dairy.** For the most part, anyway. If you have it, have just a little, and make sure it's quality cheese, aged more than 120 days (to break down the lactose).
2. **No. Gluten. Ever.** Yes, gluten is evil and will take down your health, pronto. But if you just have to have some pasta, then go with quinoa pasta—just watch your portions (the carb count on quinoa is ridiculous). Carbs break down into sugar, so excessive carbs lead to a sugar overload in your body.
3. **Legumes.** Legumes aren't allowed on the Paleo diet because they are full of lectins (read more about lectins on page 6). But if you're craving

split pea soup, go on and sprout those split peas and have 'em. I've done this. Just allow those little guys to sprout a couple of days, then make some fantabulous split pea soup. Sprouting grains and legumes destroys their lectins, making them Paleo-friendly. You're welcome.

4. **Potato patrol.** Skip the white ones and go for the purple ones, which have much more nutrition. Even so, see No. 2 regarding the quinoa pasta. Same goes for purple potatoes—go easy.

5. **Eat veggies!** Go crazy and bulk up on as many green veggies as you can, since you won't be filling up on bread and grains. Watch the starchy veggies and go with lower-glycemic stuff like broccoli, cauliflower, and, of course, dark leafy greens.

PART-TIME PALEO PRINCIPLES

As I mentioned, becoming Part-Time Paleo is about more than just what you eat. It's a lifestyle based on the following principles:

- We need to fuel our bodies with nutrients. The best source of nutrients is plants, especially organic local produce that's in season.
- Free-range eggs are packed with protein, amino acids, and minerals.
- Organic, grass-fed, pastured meat is an important protein source. Avoid consuming factory-raised animals.
- Stress-reducing activities (massage, yoga; use your imagination) are essential to good health and should be done daily.
- Exercise is important, but it should involve doing activities you enjoy.
- Rest is an often overlooked key to good health. We need to give our bodies adequate sleep so our hormones function properly.
- Fruit isn't as beneficial to the body as vegetables are. Because of its high sugar content, it should be enjoyed in small amounts.
- Nuts, berries, and seeds contain vital nutrients and should be eaten daily in moderation.

- Refined sugar, grains, legumes, gluten, and packaged, processed foods are anti-nutrient and should be avoided.
- Healthy fats like olive oil, coconut oil, grass-fed butter, and avocado do the body good.
- Vegetable oils are dangerous, man-made fats that should not be consumed by humans or any other living creature.
- Greek yogurt, kefir, and cheese aged more than 120 days are acceptable forms of dairy, if you can tolerate them. Go easy, if at all.
- Wine, especially red wine, has prebiotic properties and a great nutritional profile. It should be enjoyed in moderation.
- Counting calories is meaningless.
- Probiotics and fermented veggies are beneficial to digestion.
- Bone broth is chock-full of gut-healing properties and should become a staple in your diet.
- Be aware of your digestion and elimination.

PALEO VS. PRIMAL

You may hear the words *Paleo* and *Primal* used interchangeably, but there are some slight differences between these two diets.

Both Paleo and Primal lifestyles are based on evolutionary science that states that the diet we Westerners are eating nowadays is nothing like what our ancestors ate a hundred thousand years ago. Both the Paleo and Primal lifestyles say that if we eat what our ancestors ate, we'll be healthier.

Similarities between Paleo and Primal lifestyles include:

- Eating tons of veggies
- Eating lots of protein
- Avoiding grains
- Eliminating gluten

- Doing away with corn
- Avoiding high-fructose corn syrup
- Avoiding sugar
- Eliminating processed foods
- Enjoying the occasional wine and beer (but only gluten-free beer)
- Exercising regularly

While they are very much alike, the specific rules that differ for Paleo and Primal include the following:

- Paleoistas avoid dairy (many making an exception for grass-fed butter). Primal folks enjoy raw, fermented dairy once in a while.
- Some Paleo folks avoid saturated fats and limit their intake of fatty meats, eggs (six per day), and butter. I am not one of those folks. I eat plenty of butter, grass-fed beef, and coconut oil! Primal eaters are not afraid of saturated fats, and eggs are enjoyed freely.
- Primal allows fermented soy products and organic edamame, while Paleo has its followers avoiding soy.
- Primal allows for occasional intake of legumes, while Paleo says no.

Paleo has evolved quite a bit over the years, adopting more aspects from the Primal way of life. Many Paleoistas, for instance, eat fermented dairy and Greek yogurt. I have many Paleo pals who also don't limit the amount of eggs they eat. And lots of Paleo followers don't limit the amount of bacon that they eat either. See what I mean?

In my experience, everyone who eats this way has their own variation of a caveman-like diet and I say that's fine. The one thing that everyone agrees on is that it's real food all the time—no pseudo foods.

Rather than settle squarely in either the Paleo or the Primal camp, I have started my own: the Part-Time Paleo community.

TEN COMMON FOODS THAT SEEM PALEO BUT AREN'T

There are some foods you're going to find referenced in this book that seem perfectly nonthreatening that Paleoistas avoid as if they were junk food.

When you start eating Paleo, it's hard to wrap your mind around the fact that foods you've been led to believe are good for you are actually not, and foods you've been avoiding are actually healthy.

The basic idea of the Paleo diet is to eat foods that were available to our Paleolithic ancestors. The argument is that our physiology hasn't changed enough in the past ten thousand years to allow us to digest some of the foods that came on the scene during the onset of modern agriculture (foods like wheat).

Whole grains aren't the only "natural" foods you don't eat when you go Part-Time Paleo. The following ten foods are to be avoided:

1. **Lentils.** These little guys seem healthy enough, right? But lentils contain lectins, which are an enemy of our digestive system. You can still enjoy lentils as a Part-Time Paleoista by sprouting them to destroy the lectins. Sprout lentils the same way you would any other seed. (Read more on sprouting on page 52.)

2. **Peanuts.** Peanuts are not actually nuts; they are legumes. And legumes contain phytic acid, which binds to nutrients, preventing the body from absorbing them. Not only that, but phytic acid can lead to a leaky gut, opening the door for all kinds of problems, like autoimmune disorders and more.

3. **Rice.** Hard-core Paleoistas avoid rice, as it's a member of the cereal grain family and is essentially void of nutrients. Rice contains anti-nutrients like phytin (a form of phytic acid), which binds to minerals, making them virtually useless.

4. **Corn.** We'll go into more detail about why corn is to be avoided on page 57, but let's just say that it's almost impossible to find corn that's not GMO, and it's super high glycemic and a grain—not a vegetable! (Did I hear you gasp?)

5. **Chickpeas.** Just like peanuts, chickpeas are legumes and therefore avoided by Paleoistas.

6. **White potatoes.** White potatoes are pure starch, and as a source of nutrients, they are inferior to most other side dish options. They also belong to the nightshade family and, as such, contain chemicals called glycoalkaloids, which trigger leaky gut symptoms in folks who aren't able to tolerate them. Purple potatoes and sweet potatoes are much more nutritious options, but you need to temper your consumption with good old-fashioned moderation.

7. **Soy.** Health aficionados have eaten soy for decades. But we now know that soy is full of lectins and phytates and nonorganic soy is one of the main sources of GMOs in North America.

8. **Peas.** Green peas are legumes, so they are avoided by hard-core Paleoistas, but they aren't very harmful unless you have food sensitivities as the result of a leaky gut. Peas are quite high on the glycemic index, so if you do choose to eat them, go easy! The only exception is pea isolate. The phytates in pea isolate (like the kind in my All-in-One Smoothie Mix) are nearly eliminated in the processing and they are very easy to digest.

9. **Oats.** Cave people didn't eat oatmeal, so we don't eat oats on the Part-Time Paleo diet either. Oats contain phytic acid and should be avoided, especially if you have food sensitivities due to a leaky gut.

10. **Beans.** Again, beans are legumes and contain high amounts of lectins, so they are not Part-Time Paleo friendly.

HOW TO USE THIS BOOK

Part-Time Paleo: How to Go Paleo Without Going Crazy includes twelve weeks of menu plans to get you started (including shopping lists!). It also tells you what equipment you need in your kitchen and what ingredients you need to stock your cupboards, pantry, and fridge. In Chapter Nine, you'll find twenty Paleo freezer meals for those days you might be tempted to do takeout. There are Paleo slow cooker recipes and an entire chapter on soup. (This soup chapter, by the way, includes my fabulous Mighty Mitochondria Soup—this soup will help you get those all-important veggies in each day, deliciously.) There's a chapter about the parts of the Paleo lifestyle that I consider optional, and there's even a chapter to help you transition your children into the Part-Time Paleo lifestyle.

BEFORE YOU GO ON

Now, before you skip to the recipes, I cannot stress enough the importance of eating organic veggies, grass-fed beef, pastured pork, organic poultry, and wild fish. Whenever possible, eat as organically, locally, and in-season as you can—this ensures the high quality of your food, which in turn will deliver the highest possible amount of nutrients and phyto-nutrients to your body.

A lot of people who are considering going Paleo hesitate because they fear it will be expensive. But think about how cost effective (not to mention how much better for you) it would be to take all the cash spent on crappy food and put it toward the best food you can buy. A lot of times we end up spending more money on food that is "cheap" than we do on food that is good for us and considered expensive. When was the last time you added up what you're spending on packaged snacks and boxed cereal? How much are you spending on restaurant meals, fast food, and takeout?

When we plan our meals ahead of time, we save money because we're not throwing away wasted food that ends up rotting at the bottom of the fridge, and we're not buying items we don't need. This banked money can then be used to buy better-quality products.

Planning really is the key ingredient. Now, let's get started!

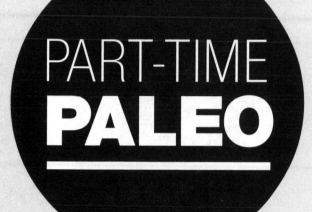

1

CHAPTER ONE

SOMETHING TO CHEW ON (WHY PALEO IS BEST FOR DIGESTION)

How much thought do you give to your digestive system? I mean, how aware are you of what happens between the time your food goes in your mouth and the time it goes out your ... well ... out of your body? Much happens along the way.

Your digestive tract is a thirty-foot-long (give or take a few feet) hollow tube running from your mouth to your rectum. Most of us think of our digestive system as nothing more than the way our food travels through our bodies, but we're forgetting a very important function of that tube.

The digestive system is tasked with more than just getting our food into our bellies. It's also responsible for protecting our bodies from toxins, chemicals, and pathogens. That big yucky tube makes up 70 percent of the body's immune system.

When your digestion is compromised, you are directly affecting your immune system. In order to have a healthy immune system, you need to have a healthy gut. You can't have one without the other.

The foods and practices followed in the Part-Time Paleo lifestyle give your system the proper elements for optimal digestion and keep out the foods that will do it harm. Make sense?

FIVE TIPS TO ENHANCE DIGESTION

1. **Chew thoroughly.** It's extremely important to the digestive process for you to chew your food.
2. **Don't drink with your meal.** Avoid drinking too much liquid with your meal because it dilutes your digestive juices. If you must drink something with a meal, drink a little water or some wine (of course). The majority of your liquid consumption, though, should be either fifteen minutes before or one hour after a meal.
3. **Stop eating when you're *almost* full.** Instead of eating until you feel full, eat only until you're *almost* full. For your foods to be broken down properly, you need to leave room for those digestive juices to do their job. You can't stuff a furnace with wood and expect to be able to start a great fire. You need some room for airflow.
4. **Consume bone broth.** With each meal, take a few ounces of bone broth, either plain or in a soup. This is a very healing food, and it will help provide you with a ton of essential nutrients—plus, eating soup (like my delicious Mighty Mitochondria Soup) fills you up and helps you meet your nutritional quota for veggies in a very enjoyable way.
5. **Eat fermented foods.** Fermented foods such as kimchi and sauerkraut should be eaten frequently because that fermentation sends good bacteria to the gut, helping in the process of digestion. You can make your own fermented vegetables quite easily.

CHEW, CHEW, CHEW

The more time your food and your saliva spend together, the better. Contact with saliva not only makes it easier for food to go through the esophagus, but that saliva is also full of enzymes that play a role in the chemical process of digesting our food. The first stage of fat digestion actually happens in the mouth.

Your saliva starts breaking down the food you put into your mouth, and from there, the food continues to break down until it's reduced to minuscule particles that your cells will use for energy, repair, and ongoing maintenance.

Chewing food slowly and taking time to actually taste and savor every bite goes a long way toward enjoying each morsel you put in your mouth—*and* it helps give your digestive process the time it needs with your saliva. We eat so quickly that we don't give our food the attention it needs from our saliva for proper nutrient absorption.

When we chew our food properly, large food molecules are broken down into smaller particles, giving our food a larger surface area as it goes through the digestive system. This breaking up of food molecules is essential to good digestion. It's also easier on your esophagus to swallow smaller pieces of food.

When your food isn't chewed up well, the fragments are too large to be broken down properly. Nutrients aren't extracted from the food like they should be, leading to undigested food, which encourages bacterial overgrowth in the colon. (Can you say flatulence?)

Another useful side effect of chewing each bite more than once or twice is that it slows down the entire process of eating a meal, giving your belly and your brain the message that you're full much sooner, which prevents you from overeating.

Now, I'm not going to tell you to chew each bite fifty times, but a good rule of thumb is to chew until you can't tell what kind of food you're eating anymore based on texture. For example, if you're eating an apple, don't stop chewing until you can't tell the peel from the flesh of the apple.

The digestive system is responsible for getting all those bits and pieces to the proper places within the body, while also getting rid of everything that needs to be eliminated along the way—toxins, pathogens, and other nasties. Your job is to put the highest-quality foods possible into that system. One could argue that the digestive process technically starts with the items in your grocery bags. The more organic foods you put into your mouth, the easier a job you're giving your digestive system, since it won't have as many chemicals to sort through.

THE POWER OF PROBIOTICS

One often overlooked aspect of good gut health is getting plenty of those good bacteria moving through your system. I'm talking about probiotics.

Good gut bacteria are extremely beneficial to your health. Did you know that there are roughly 450 different species of bacteria sitting in your gastrointestinal tract right now? If you put all of those little critters on a kitchen scale, they'd add up to about three pounds! Now, I don't know about you, but that seems like a significant enough population to be concerned about.

We need to be sure that at least 85 percent of those bacteria are in the helpful court—the probiotic side of the equation. Those probiotics activate T cells (the cancer fighters) and trigger many immune system reactions throughout your entire body. And when you consider that about 70 percent of your immune system lives right there in your gut, don't you think it's smart to be feeding your gut what it needs to maintain your health?

Your body is counting on 15 percent or less of your intestinal flora to be pathogenic, so it's up to you to do what you can to keep things optimally balanced, and probiotics are a terrific way to improve your balance. You will find probiotic capsules and powders (I prefer the capsules) at your local health food store or in the health food section of most well-stocked grocery stores (look in the refrigerated section).

Some of the benefits of probiotics include:

- **Reversal of ulcers.** Probiotics may actually reverse irritable bowl syndrome, ulcerative colitis, Crohn's disease, and ulcers. If you've had a gut inflammation of any kind, start taking probiotics ASAP.
- **Immunity boost.** Probiotics may help prevent colds, allergies, and flu.
- **Better breast milk.** If pregnant women and nursing mothers take

probiotics, Mom's breast milk has enhanced immune protection for baby.

- **Relief from GS symptoms.** If you're suffering from gluten sensitivity (GS) or celiac symptoms, you may find relief if you add probiotics to your diet.
- **Beat the yeast.** A healthy balance of probiotics in the system may help prevent yeast infections.
- **Cancer prevention.** Probiotics help to nourish certain enzymes in the body, which may go on to reduce tumor production in your body.
- **Fight bad foods.** If you eat any nonorganic meat or processed foods containing GMOs, you are likely consuming antibiotics. Eating these foods kills healthy bacteria in the gut, so consuming probiotics may help to restore your gut's healthy balance.

There is some evidence to suggest that probiotics can help those affected by autism. A doctor by the name of Natasha Campbell-McBride moved her son off the autism spectrum by restoring healthy probiotic levels in his body, thereby relieving inflammation in his body. The diet she developed is known as the GAPS (Gut and Psychology Syndrome) diet, and it is followed widely throughout the United States and Canada.

So, how do you get all the probiotics you need?

Well, first off, you can take a supplement. This is absolutely crucial if you've been on antibiotics, which kill healthy bacteria in your gut. I wish more doctors would recommend that patients take a probiotic while on a round of antibiotics, but I digress.

Wholesome foods are always preferable over supplements. I'm a big believer in eating fermented foods, which are essentially probiotics! Keep on reading to find a fermented food primer, and learn to make these magical foods yourself on pages 10–13.

A healthy digestive system will get the bad stuff out while hanging on to the good stuff. If you're digesting food properly, you will feel fantastic, get sick infrequently, and live longer and, God willing, disease-free.

Doing your part for your digestive system means that you have to eat real foods. Those real foods must be quality foods, like organic produce, grass-fed meats, and free-range, pastured poultry and eggs.

The fake foods, sugar, and pesticides found in the Standard American Diet wreak havoc on the human body, jeopardizing our very health. Our bodies do not recognize this stuff as food, and consequently, they are not digested well. This also goes for legumes and grains—foods that were introduced by the onset of modern agriculture. They are tough on the system and can actually cause significant damage to your gut. Much of this can be blamed on dietary lectins.

THE SCOOP ON DIETARY LECTINS

Dietary lectins are probably not on your radar. Most everyday folks don't know about lectins, and neither do many doctors. Considering the damage these nasty little sons of guns can do, that's really not good.

Lectins are proteins that bind to carbohydrates, cells, and tissues. These proteins do not break down easily. They cause inflammation in the body, they can be toxic, and they are resistant to digestive enzymes. Think of them as invisible thorns ripping you up on the inside.

This resistance to stomach acid means that lectins are free to latch on to the wall of your stomach, where they can then contribute to the erosion of your intestinal barrier. That, my friend, is known as leaky gut, and it's about as pretty as it sounds.

When the gut lining is damaged, other proteins can sneak through into the body in an undigested state, causing all kinds of problems, including:

- Colitis
- Crohn's disease
- Irritable bowel syndrome (IBS)
- Celiac sprue

- Insulin-dependent diabetes
- Rheumatoid arthritis
- Ulcers
- Food allergies and sensitivities
- Low energy
- Weight gain

When lectins circulate through your bloodstream, they're then free to bind to any tissue in your body, including the pancreas, the thyroid, and even the collagen in your joints. Your white blood cells attack the tissue that the lectin has attached to, effectively destroying it. Lectin protein in wheat, for example, is known to cause rheumatoid arthritis, as it attaches to joint collagen.

And lectins are found in a lot of the food we eat, including:

- Legumes
- Dairy
- Grains: wheat, wheat germ, rice, oats, buckwheat, rye, barley, corn, millet, and quinoa
- Nightshade foods: tomatoes, potatoes, cucumbers, eggplant, and peppers
- Some seafood

Some people do seem to be able to tolerate lectins better than others, and that's because they have the ideal balance of beneficial flora and a strong immune system.

WHY ARE PURPLE POTATOES BETTER THAN WHITE?

There's no nutrition to speak of in a plate of starchy white potatoes, so we avoid white tubers when we eat Part-Time Paleo. Purple potatoes, however, are a different story, and they make a great stand-in for your old familiar spuds.

Purple potatoes were first grown in Peru, where thousands of years ago they were eaten only by Incan kings because they were so valuable.

You can now find hundreds of varieties of purple potatoes in the United States, and they are not reserved for royalty! The darker their color, the greater the antioxidant content within those potato skins.

Purple potatoes contain iron, folic acid, vitamin C, and potassium. The darkest of them actually have as much antioxidant power as spinach, kale, and brussels sprouts.

While they are a little lower on the glycemic index, they're not without their carb problems. Keeping carbs on the low side keeps inflammation (and your weight) down.

Then there are some folks with severe lectin sensitivity. Symptoms of severe lectin intolerance include:

- Memory impairment
- Sleep problems
- Irregular moods
- Gas
- Swollen joints
- Water retention
- Constipation and/or diarrhea
- Fatigue
- Hives
- Headaches

If you're in this category, your body is unable to stop lectins from binding to cells, and you must eliminate lectins from your diet if you want to feel better.

Most people think they're getting along fine until they eliminate wheat, dairy, and nightshades from their diet and feel the benefits firsthand with improved energy, better sleep, and a better overall feeling of well-being. With your Part-Time Paleo lifestyle, you're about to discover these benefits yourself.

FERMENTED FOODS: A PRIMER

I think our ancestors would be pretty surprised at how fermented foods seem to have all but disappeared from our diets.

Since ancient times, humans around the world have been fermenting their food before eating or drinking it. Wine was being made at least eight thousand years ago. Milk fermentation has been happening since around 3000 BC, and folks were eating leavened bread around 1500 BC.

Our grandmothers made sauerkraut and pickles via lacto-fermentation (using salt), whereas today we use vinegar. They used wild yeast (sourdough) to leaven their bread. Those types of fermentation provided us with probiotics, replenishing the good bacteria in our bodies.

Today, almost everything we eat is pasteurized. We use antibacterial soap and drink chlorinated water. We take antibiotic drugs. These modern "fixes" have left us with an imbalanced level of bacteria in our guts, and that can fuel illness.

Adding fermented foods to your diet will help restore those levels of healthy bacteria, and it will do wonders for your well-being.

Here are some good reasons to eat fermented foods:

- **Improved digestion.** Eating fermented foods is sort of like having it already partially digested before it hits your stomach, because the food has been processed and broken down by acids. That allows your body to take the good out of the food without doing as much heavy lifting. When you improve digestion, nutrient absorption is naturally improved as well.
- **Vitamin boost.** When you ferment food, you boost its vitamin content, especially with fermented dairy products like kefir.
- **Gut health.** You need good bacteria in your gut to avoid yeast infections, irritable bowel syndrome, constipation, gluten intolerance, lactose intolerance, and lots of other nasty things. Eating fermented foods can help strike the right balance.

- **Flavor.** Why does sauerkraut taste so good on our sausages and corned beef go so well with pickles? Because they're delicious, that's why! Fermented foods are healthy and delicious.

Fermenting food is inexpensive, requires very basic ingredients (salt and mason jars), and helps to preserve foods for a long period of time.

To get more fermented foods into your diet, drink kombucha (a fermented tea you'll find in Asian markets) or kefir. Eat naturally fermented condiments that you buy at the store, or make your own at home. Kimchi, sauerkraut, salsa, and pickles are all examples of fermented condiments you can easily make yourself.

PART-TIME PALEO FERMENTED RECIPES

Jalapeño-Peach Salsa

Yields approx. 3 cups

> 2 cups peeled and chopped peaches
> ½ cup chopped red onion
> 1 clove garlic, pressed
> 2 tablespoons minced jalapeño
> 2 tablespoons lemon juice
> 2 teaspoons sea salt
> 2 tablespoons purified water, as needed

Combine peaches, onion, garlic, jalapeño, lemon juice, and sea salt in a bowl and mix well. Transfer to a canning jar and, using a spoon, crush the mixture to release as much liquid as possible. Liquid should cover the mixture to prevent mold. If you do not have enough liquid, add just enough water to make sure mixture is covered (you may not use the entire 2 tablespoons). Leave at least an inch between the salsa and the top of the jar, as it will expand as it ferments. Cover tightly and store in a warm place for 2–5 days. Taste periodically, and when the salsa suits your taste, transfer to the fridge. Chill and enjoy.

Cranberry Mango Chutney

Yields approx. 4 cups

- 2 cups chopped bing cherries
- 1 cup fresh cranberries
- 1 cup peeled and chopped mango
- ½ teaspoon ground cloves
- ½ teaspoon grated ginger
- ¼ teaspoon ground cardamom
- 2 tablespoons lime juice
- 1 teaspoon sea salt
- 2 tablespoons purified water, as needed

Combine cherries, cranberries, mangoes, cloves, ginger, cardamom, lime juice, and sea salt in a bowl and mix well. Transfer to a canning jar and, using a spoon, crush the mixture to release as much liquid as possible. Liquid should cover the mixture to prevent mold. If you do not have enough liquid, add just enough water to make sure mixture is covered (you may not use the entire 2 tablespoons). Leave at least an inch between the chutney and the top of the jar, as it will expand as it ferments. Cover tightly and store in a warm place for 2–5 days. Taste periodically, and when the chutney suits your taste, transfer to the fridge. Chill and enjoy.

Sweet and Spicy Apricot Date Chutney

Yields approx. 3 cups

- 2 cups peeled and chopped apricots
- ½ cup diced yellow onion

½ cup chopped dates

½ teaspoon freshly ground pepper

½ teaspoon dried thyme

1 teaspoon dried crushed rosemary

2 tablespoons honey

1 tablespoon cider vinegar

2 tablespoons lemon juice

1 tablespoon sea salt

2 tablespoons purified water, as needed

Combine apricots, onion, dates, pepper, thyme, and rosemary in a bowl and mix well. In a small saucepan over low heat, combine honey, vinegar, lemon juice, and sea salt, and heat through, but do not reduce. Cool and pour over apricot mixture. Stir well, transfer to a canning jar, and, using a spoon, crush the mixture to release as much liquid as possible. Liquid should cover the mixture to prevent mold. If you do not have enough liquid, add just enough water to make sure mixture is covered. Leave at least an inch between the chutney and the top of the jar, as it will expand as it ferments. Cover tightly and store in a warm place for 2–5 days. Taste periodically, and when the chutney suits your taste, transfer to the fridge. Chill and enjoy.

Fermented Dill Pickles and Pearl Onions

Yields approx. 4–5 cups

2 tablespoons mustard seeds

3 tablespoons dried dill

3 cloves garlic, pressed

½ cup chopped white onion

3 cups pickling cucumbers, sliced ¼ inch thick

1 cup pearl onions, peeled

2 tablespoons sea salt

1 cup purified water

Place mustard seeds, dill, garlic, and white onion in a large mason jar. Place sliced cucumbers and pearl onions on top. Mix sea salt and water until salt is dissolved, and pour into the jar. Add more water if pickles are not covered, but be sure to leave at least an inch between the liquid and the top of the jar. Seal the jar, and store for 2 days at room temperature. Taste pickles, and when desired flavor is reached, seal tightly and refrigerate.

Spiced Maple Baby Carrots

Yields approx. 1–2 quarts

1 (16 oz) bag baby carrots
1 tablespoon orange zest
1 teaspoon lime zest
1 teaspoon lemon zest
2 teaspoons grated ginger
1 teaspoon ground cinnamon
¼ teaspoon cardamom
3 tablespoons pure maple syrup
2 tablespoons sea salt
1 cup purified water, plus more as needed

Place carrots in a large mason jar. In a separate container, combine orange, lime, and lemon zests with ginger, cinnamon, cardamom, maple syrup, sea salt, and water. Stir until salt is dissolved, and pour over carrots. Add more purified water to cover carrots, leaving an inch between the liquid and the top of the jar. Seal tightly and store at room temperature for 3–7 days, until carrots reach desired flavor. Then reseal tightly, refrigerate, and enjoy!

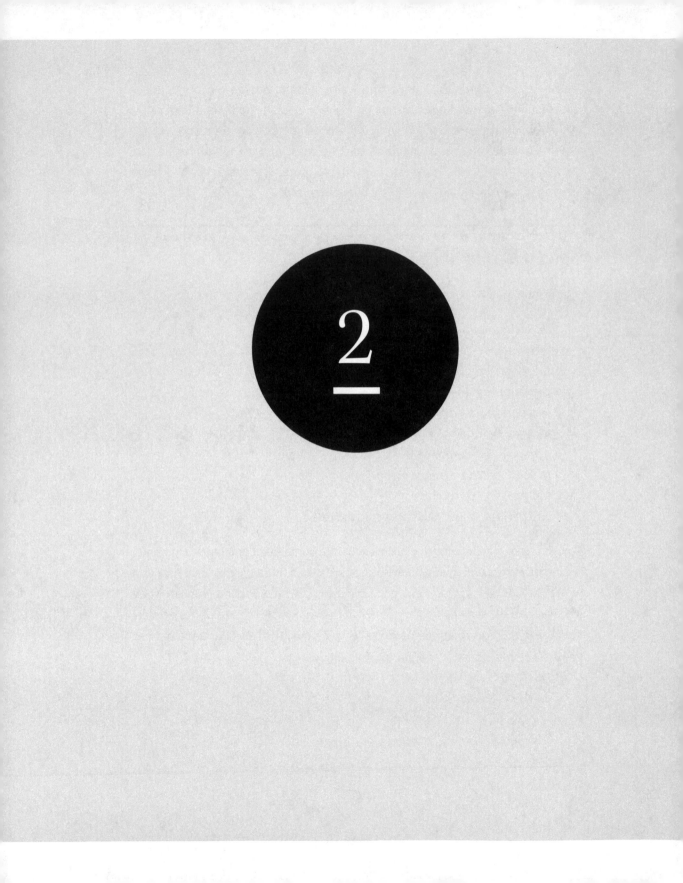

CHAPTER TWO
THE PART-TIME PALEO LIFESTYLE

I've learned a lot since I embarked on my Paleo journey. For instance, I've learned I'll never be a CrossFitter (one WOD was more than enough—if you don't know what that is, that's okay; you don't want to); I'll never wear Vibrams (peep toes are more my style than shoes with toes); and I promise you, pemmican will never cross my lips (it's made with dried meat, rendered fat, and, if you're lucky, some dried berries). I struggle with eating animal innards and will even admit to gagging on liver. I'm hardly the paragon of a Paleo warrior.

For a while, I felt guilty about it. I tried all of the above (okay, all except the Vibrams), but I just couldn't force myself to continue with them. I mean, if I can't even stand the smell of liver, what makes me think that I'd do better with less mainstream innards like pancreas or brain? The very idea is nauseating to me. I can't do it, so I can't tell you to. It's disingenuous and just plain wrong—not my style.

So, where does that leave me and my tribe, people like me who haven't followed the Paleo prescribed way of life to the letter but still firmly embrace the sound nutritional principles of Paleo that work for them?

Welcome to the Part-Time Paleo world, where Vibrams are optional and you don't ever have to set foot in a CrossFit warehouse if you don't want to.

The Part-Time Paleo lifestyle is a hybrid of sorts. You don't have to worry if you haven't spent time growing or fermenting your own foods. You don't have to do (or be) it all to get great results. The Part-Time Paleo lifestyle is one that optimizes nutrition but doesn't make you feel guilty if you throw a sprinkle of good cheese on that soup on occasion. You do as well as you can the majority of the time so that you don't gasp in horror if your child eats cake at a birthday party.

Life happens. We live in a non-Paleo world—you know that. (Just go to the grocery store if you need the reality check.) We cannot be so dogmatic in everything we do that we alienate those we love and care about. Some people become such hard-core Paleoistas that they turn off everyone around them. Now, that doesn't mean throwing your diet to the wind when you visit family or go out to dinner; it just means you may need to make a tiny adjustment every now and again. If doing so compromises your health (because you have celiac disease or an allergy to dairy or some other issue), then, obviously, don't put yourself in jeopardy. Likewise, if eating something makes you feel bad and achy all over, you simply can explain that you have an allergy and you're sorry, but no—all said with a smile on your face and the ability to change the subject quickly to the weather or sports or even politics. Nothing can be quite as polarizing as what one eats.

I know you're probably used to books with rigid diet rules, and yes, there are rules for following the Paleo diet, but with the Part-Time Paleo diet, you're given a dash of latitude to use at will.

I've found that saying "you can never eat this again" is akin to double-dog daring someone to eat it. It makes the forbidden look tempting and leaves it constantly on your mind. Dreams of sourdough loaves dancing in your head . . . been there, done that.

So my solution is quite simple: Rather than dogmatic statements ("I'll never eat bread again"), I say, "If I want to feel my best and protect my thyroid and health, I choose not to eat that bread." I understand the difference between eating for health and eating for entertainment. Interestingly, the further into this journey I go, the less willing I am to take the risk. It's easier to stay with my diet than to veer off. At a family barbecue, my hamburger is naked, I skip the baked beans, and I double up on the salad. I'll usually skip the dessert, but if someone makes home-made ice cream, I might have a bite or two. To me, that's worth it. Ice cream from the store? Not so much. Make sense?

BUT WHAT IF I'M INVITED TO DINNER?

If I'm invited to a dinner party, I politely let my hosts know I have gluten intolerance. That problem is, thankfully, quite common and never an issue. Now, if I went to a dinner party and said, "I don't eat gluten, legumes, beans, or dairy," I could leave my hostess bewildered and wish-ing she hadn't invited me. So for me, I am sure to avoid the food that is the most problematic—gluten. I stay away from it 99.9 percent of the time. Dairy for one meal will not make me feel bad like gluten will, so I avoid my biggest enemy and forget about the rest for one meal.

Now, some people cannot do this and need to stay 100 percent com-pliant with the diet or risk a health crisis. I know a few people like that. My suggestion is that you let the hostess know about your limitations and offer to bring something. Actually, you should insist, and while you're at it, don't forget to bring a stellar gift to make up for the fact that your hostess will likely be stressed on your behalf for the entire party.

There is such a thing as a Part-Time Paleo lifestyle. I am living it. Being Part-Time Paleo elevates my life on many levels: work, play, and just flat-out enjoyment.

THE PART-TIME PALEO LIFESTYLE

So, what does a Part-Time Paleo lifestyle look like? Well, first up is exercise. Three days a week, I work out at a gym for an hour—half of that time is spent in weight lifting and the other half in interval aerobic training. If I'm in town and really want to move the needle (as in, the needle on the scale), I'll try to add another day.

For me, the ritual of leaving the house, working out, and coming home is worth the inconvenience of having to drive. It's an appointment I keep with myself (unless I'm traveling), and I redeem that time listening to CDs I wouldn't otherwise have the time to listen to; it's a total win-win.

I've also developed a fondness for yoga and find this discipline of stretching and deep breathing not only a thorough stress reliever but also a great way to keep my muscles from being overly sore.

And lastly, I've joined one of those places where you can get a massage once a month for less than fifty dollars. At first I thought it was just a little too indulgent getting a massage once a month. But after studying stress and its effects on the body, I rejected the mind-set of it being a big extravagance and instead began to think of it as something I do for my health and well-being. I must admit, it's made all the difference in the world.

PALEOISTAS SAY . . . RELAX!

When your body senses that it's under some sort of stress—physical or psychological—powerful hormones are released into your bloodstream. Our caveman ancestors needed this to happen back in the days when they had to count on a burst of adrenaline to help them fight or outrun a saber-toothed tiger.

I'm going out on a limb here to say that your stress isn't directly related to a saber-toothed tiger. But guess what? Your body is still releasing those same hormones. While you're experiencing that adrenaline rush, your body releases cortisol, a hormone that sends a signal that energy stores are being depleted. That signal tells the body to replenish those energy stores because outrunning a tiger uses up lots of calories.

But when you're stressed and you're not actually fleeing or fighting to burn calories, when your body is told to replenish energy, you get hungry. You get very hungry. And for as long as your body experiences stress, you continue to pump cortisol through your veins, getting hungrier and hungrier.

When we feel that stress hunger, we're not reaching for carrot sticks and apples. We end up craving sweet, fatty, salty foods because our brains know those foods help release our pleasure chemicals, which help us to feel less tense. Those sweet and salty foods give us such a feeling of euphoria that our brains become addicted to them. When we feel anxious or stressed, we keep reaching for those foods.

That constant release of cortisol slows down the production of testosterone, a hormone that builds muscle. With less testosterone, you have less muscle mass, and muscle mass burns calories. So even if you are able to resist those cravings, you are still in an unhealthy scenario. As if that weren't bad enough, cortisol encourages the body to hold on to fat.

Stress is not a laughing matter. Part-Time Paleo means taking time out to relax. It's key to this lifestyle.

Yoga and a monthly massage work for my budget and lifestyle.

EXERCISE

So, let's talk about exercise for a moment. I think a lot of people believe it has to hurt a lot and take up a lot of time in order to be effective. I deliberately spend an hour on exercise three to four times a week (plus yoga when I can), but it's a personal preference that works for my lifestyle.

But for those who have no time, there's a way to get your exercise done in as little as four minutes. Yes, four minutes and only four times a week. It's called Tabata training, named for Japanese researcher Dr. Izumi Tabata, who found that the quickest possible route to fitness is with twenty-second intervals, ten-second rests, and eight rounds of training. It's tough, quick, and dirty.

A typical Tabata training session might look like this: twenty seconds each of squats, sit-ups, push-ups, and triceps dips with ten-second rests in between. You do one exercise, rest, move to the next exercise, rest, and so on until you've completed all four exercises. That is one set—just seven more and you're done in less than five minutes. You can do all of those exercises right now in your living room, with no equipment. See how easy it is? Check out YouTube for tons of free Tabata training videos.

I mentioned yoga as well as a viable option for exercise. With the exception of hot yoga (I'm not a fan—it makes me claustrophobic—but a lot of folks love it, so it might be something for you to try), I find yoga to be an incredible stress reliever, and it is one of the wisest ways to stay young and healthy, regardless of age. Strength, flexibility, and balance are three key components to fitness, and you get all three of these factors at work when you practice yoga.

SLEEP. SLEEP. SLEEP.

Early humans did hard, grueling work all day long—well, as long as the sun shone. They were busy building shelters, making clothes, and hunting and growing food. When the sun went down, they most likely spent time playing simple games or making babies. Then it was time to sleep.

Our lives don't quite work that way anymore. Most Americans don't get enough sleep. We're go, go, go all the time. And this sleep deprivation is not good for our health. Lack of sleep puts you at risk for high blood pressure, heart disease, diabetes, heart attack, stroke, and even heart failure.

Have you ever heard of circadian rhythm? Your circadian rhythm is a cycle of chemical and physical processes that your body undergoes each day in response to light. This rhythm is quite dependent upon your body's daily exposure to light versus dark. Not sleeping when it's dark affects that circadian rhythm, leading to depression, weight gain, poor energy, and all kinds of other miserable side effects.

With circadian rhythm, the body's levels of cortisol and melatonin fluctuate. You might remember that cortisol acts as a stimulant. Melatonin is a hormone that makes you sleepy.

When your circadian rhythm is running along tickety-boo, your cortisol levels are high in the morning, and in the evening when it gets dark, your melatonin kicks in to make you sleepy.

When you feel sleepy in the evening and you don't give in to that drowsiness, your body has to make more cortisol to keep you awake. All that cortisol keeps your body in a stress state, which, if we remember, leads to all kinds of unhealthy issues, including weight gain.

Good sleep patterns are necessary for almost all hormonal functioning within the human body. Some hormones simply can't function at all without sleep. One key hormone, for example, is leptin, which is responsible for your appetite, your immune system, and your metabolism. Leptin is controlled through sleep cycles.

Listen to your body! Make sleep a priority in your life. Combine it with a stress-reducing activity such as taking a nice warm epsom salt bath before bed. Use a white noise machine or buy darkening shades for your bedroom. Do whatever it takes, but protect your sleep.

CAFFEINE: FRIEND OR FOE?

Caffeine is a drug found in coffee, tea, soft drinks, energy drinks, and chocolate, and a lot of people have quite a solid relationship with at least one of these items. I very much enjoy my coffee, so I can relate to any of you with dependence issues!

The question is . . . is caffeine a friend or a foe?

I'm not going to tell you that caffeine should be avoided altogether, so don't worry about that. Coffee is great, but let's look at some information about the effects caffeine has on the human body, and then you can go ahead and draw your own conclusions from there.

Ever wonder why you feel the effects of caffeine in your system so quickly? It's because it goes straight to your hormones and stays in your system for hours. Once you've ingested it, caffeine causes the following hormonal responses:

- **Adrenaline rush.** Caffeine gives you that adrenaline rush that perks you up. It puts you in fight-or-flight mode so that your body is sitting there at your desk on edge, waiting for something to respond to. That state will end up leaving you tired later on so that you need more coffee to bring you out of the doldrums. From there, you'll be jumpy and agitated, reaching for more caffeine or sugar to make you feel good.

- **Adenosine inhibition.** Adenosine is a hormone that calms your body, and caffeine inhibits its absorption. That's why you feel alert just after you drink a coffee and why you sometimes can't sleep for even hours afterward.

- **Increased cortisol.** Caffeine makes your body create more cortisol, which, as we have discussed already, is also known as the stress hormone. When you have too much cortisol in your system, you end up moody, but you can also gain weight or develop heart disease or even diabetes.

- **Increased dopamine.** When you consume caffeine, your body will increase its levels of dopamine, giving you the same sort of feeling as if you were using amphetamines. That makes you feel happy for a little while, but when the buzz wears off, you feel worse than you did before.

Now, caffeine isn't *all* bad.

While it can lead to weight gain because of increased cortisol levels (which can also, again, make you crave fatty, sugary carbs), some research suggests that caffeine can speed up your metabolism. If you consume caffeine before exercise, it can also help your body break down fat more efficiently. If you combine your morning coffee with exercise, for example, it may help enhance your performance, and you'll have a boost from the exercise that will help negate any slump in your mood from the effects of the caffeine wearing off.

What Does This Tell Us?

Caffeine can be a friend if you take it in small, controlled doses. You also may want to stop ingesting caffeine after 2:00 P.M.

When you buy coffee, I recommend buying organic fair trade beans and grinding them yourself. This ensures you get the freshest coffee possible because the oil in coffee beans causes ground coffee to go rancid quite quickly. The type of water you use (tap versus filtered) can also affect the taste of your java! Brew your coffee with filtered water for the best-tasting cup.

Cutting Down

If you have a major caffeine addiction, you can experience serious withdrawal symptoms when you try to cut back, such as headaches or irritability. To negate those nasty effects, be sure to drink lots of water to help flush excess caffeine from your body. As you try to cut out the caffeine, start mixing it with decaffeinated versions (so mix coffee with decaf or black tea with herbal). As a general rule, if you drink more than a couple of cups of java a day, you might want to consider drinking half-regular and half-decaf—organic, please!

Use a water-processed decaf coffee, too, because you don't need any extra chemicals.

Paleo purists generally try to get a solid nine hours of sleep per night. Sounds blissful, doesn't it? As an added bonus to getting all that sleep, when your sleep cycle is running optimally, you won't need to set an alarm clock anymore because your body will naturally wake you up in the morning.

How hard will it be to get on board with a lifestyle that celebrates bacon, butter, massage, moderate exercise, and restful sleep? Not hard at all. But first we need to get your kitchen equipped.

3

CHAPTER THREE

EQUIPPING YOUR KITCHEN

One of the most important elements in pursuing a Paleo lifestyle is making sure you and your kitchen have a good working relationship. Food is at the core of all good health, and you can't eat good food without first procuring, storing, preparing, and ultimately cooking it.

Your kitchen has to be set up with the proper equipment, the workspace needs to accommodate your needs, and the food requires proper storage to make it all happen.

I've witnessed firsthand how an ill-equipped kitchen can ruin even the best of intentions. I've read many a sob story from my friends and customers who have a difficult time pulling it all together on the kitchen front. In my experience, this malady all too often stems from an unorganized space with too many tchotchkes on the counters. The cupboards are stuffed to overflowing with fifteen-year-old wedding presents that have never been used and way too many storage containers that no longer have corresponding lids.

Here's a short and easy quiz to find out if your kitchen is workable:

1. Are there matchy-matchy canisters sitting on your countertops still holding the flour, sugar, and coffee you put in them in 2003?
2. Is there a bread maker, pasta maker, or some other small appliance taking up residence in that precious space that you have zero need for?
3. When you open the cupboard that holds your storage containers, do they come flying out to greet you each and every time?

If you answered yes to any one of these questions, then it is definitely time to do a massive declutter and clean up your kitchen. You're going to need that space, and you're also going to need the proper equipment to streamline your kitchen experience. This one step can be revolutionary.

Why do we work so hard at not spending any time in the kitchen? We look for shortcuts, convenience, and ease. I love shortcuts as much as the next cook, but I also believe there's pleasure to be found in a meal well prepared.

We're not a lazy lot, but we've been sold a bill of goods. We've been so beholden to saving time that we've embraced all of the mass-produced processed ingredients, which in turn begat some culinary creations like a casserole made with a can of soup and the like.

What started as a loving and nurturing task was hijacked by the food industry, which now sells inferior food (if you could even call it "food").

Most people consider food preparation to be drudgery (or worse). And yet this daily task is such a powerful thing if you think about it correctly. In your very hands, the food you buy with the good money you earned can completely transform your health and the health of your family. It's a total power trip, really: to be able to prepare food that will alter the course of your health, food that can change your destiny.

Food is, as Hippocrates said so many centuries ago, medicine. So let's all adopt that attitude and make those kitchens sacred spaces that we can honor with our presence, our food, and ultimately our dearest loved ones as we bring them to the family dinner table.

An easy way to make your kitchen workable is to start knowing you'll need an adequate workspace—cooking is going to be happening here, and lots of it. Make the best of what you've got. No comparing your kitchen to anyone else's—that's a waste of time and energy. Clear the counters as best you can, leaving only what you truly use. For me, that's the coffeemaker, Blendtec blender, and slow cooker. I have a nice big kitchen with a large island as well, and I could afford to be a little more extravagant with decorating my kitchen space and putting out more "stuff," but I refrain. This is my domain, a beloved workspace, a place where I lovingly prepare the food my family and friends are going to enjoy. I enjoy preparing it all the more if my space is clean and organized. Once you've defined order in your own kitchen, it's time to get some equipment in there so you can get busy.

PART-TIME PALEO KITCHEN ESSENTIALS

- **Good knives.** I'm pretty persnickety about knives, as they are the primary culinary tools in the kitchen. Everyone needs a couple of basics: a French knife or Santoku and a paring knife. If this were all you had, you could get by. All the chopping will be done with your French knife (or Santoku, my personal fave); the paring knife will, well, pare. Nice to have, but not completely necessary, are a slicing or carving knife for the epic roasts you'll be making and a serrated blade to cut tomatoes. (Notice the bread knife is missing from the lineup!) You don't even need the serrated blade if you have a stone to sharpen your knives and keep them as sharp as a sous chef's; all you have to do is sharpen them every time you use them, which is easy enough.

- **Microplane.** You should be able to find a microplane at your local big box store if you don't have a kitchen store nearby. This inexpensive grating tool can be used to zest a lemon or lime and to finely grate some nutmeg or even a bit of dark chocolate.
- **Garlic press.** Mincing garlic results in a sticky, stinky mess on your fingers. I'm all about getting the job done with a garlic press.
- **Graduated mixing bowls.** Every Paleoista needs a graduated set of stainless steel bowls. Use the small one for whisking eggs, the medium one for tossing together an impromptu coleslaw, and the big one for whipping up a meatloaf.
- **Measuring cups.** You need a set of dry measuring cups and a liquid measuring cup. While both can measure a half cup of something, the measurement is off if you use the liquid measuring cup for dry ingredients and vice versa. For reference: The liquid measuring cup is the one with the spout, and the dry measuring cups are the little scoop-like nesting cups.
- **Kitchen shears.** I have two pairs of kitchen shears and I use them all the time. One is for things like cutting up chicken and bacon; the other is for chopping herbs and canned tomatoes (you put the shears in the can and ship away!) and trimming artichoke leafs.
- **Kitchen tongs.** I use kitchen tongs for all sorts of things, from turning meat to making garlicky sautéed spinach and greens.
- **Copper-bottomed stainless cookware.** I love big skillets and lovely sauté pans with sloped sides. I have both and use them constantly. Both serve purposes large and small, and you need an assortment of sizes. I promise you will use them regularly, so don't shy away from owning a few.
- **Soup pots.** Go big or go home. If you make gigantic batches of freezable soups and stews, you'll never be wanting.
- **Saucepans.** You're going to need a stack of saucepans in graduated sizes (just like the mixing bowls) for a variety of jobs, large and small.

LEARN TO LOVE YOUR SLOW COOKER AND YOUR BLENDER

I mentioned the slow cooker earlier. Slow cookers are amazing in a Paleo or Part-Time Paleo kitchen. These are the small appliances that will create all those nutrient-dense bone broths you will come to love, along with delicious stews and tremendous soups. You'll also appreciate the versatility of this fine machine in the depth of summer, when the idea of heating up the oven is positively reprehensible. A slow cooker can stand in to slowly "bake" something like a sweet potato or a layered veggie dish that would normally require turning on the oven.

The Blendtec is a personal favorite of mine, as my morning smoothie is my favorite Part-Time Paleo departure. Full disclosure here: I have my own special protein blend and mix (you can find more information about my All-in-One Smoothie Mix and FiberMender at the end of this book, in the Resources section), and there is (gasp) some pea protein in there! It's pea isolate, though, and it doesn't give you gas or make your tummy hurt like a lot of legumes do. I use my Blendtec to make my smoothie nearly every morning. I have chocolate-, vanilla-, and chai-flavored protein mixes, so the variety and flavors are endlessly delicious. I'm never bored, and I absolutely adore the ease of getting all that nutrition in a glass before heading out the door.

In addition to making smoothies every morning, my Blendtec is a workhorse and gets "cream" soups made in a jiffy. It also makes Paleo mayo, nut butters, and more. For years, I could never understand why anyone would pay that kind of money for a blender (mine cost $400) when you can pick up a pretty cute-looking one at any box store for less than fifty dollars. Then I owned one. The rest is history. Seriously, you need a good blender. If not a Blendtec, then something with at least nine hundred watts of power. The Blendtec can go 240 miles an hour. It's pretty much the NASCAR champ of the blender series. I strongly recommend it.

If you want more information on setting up your kitchen and some fun "show-and-tell," I've set up special videos and resources just for you on my book website.[*]

---

[*] http://www.parttimepaleobook.com

CHAPTER FOUR

A PALEO PRIMER: HOW TO STOCK YOUR PANTRY, FRIDGE, AND FREEZER

I've been at this for a few years, and stocking pantries, fridges, and freezers is a specialty of mine. I'm sure I've worn out my own mantra by now—"a well-stocked pantry is a cook's best friend"—but honestly, isn't it the truth? How fun and easy is it to go to your pantry, fridge, or freezer and be able to snag what you need to make an amazing dinner without having to run to the grocery store for a missing ingredient?

Diligent pantry stocking isn't something you do "just in case." It's something you turn into a weekly habit because *this* is the food that will feed you, comfort you, and help you feed your family with minimal stress. Not having what you need necessitates endless trips to the grocery store and wastes gas and time.

Having and maintaining a pantry that serves you and your family is a definite skill set everyone needs to master. (Pssst . . . you can go online[*] and get this same Basic Paleo Pantry Stock-Up List, but in a downloadable and printable format.)

The basics for any good Part-Time Paleo pantry, fridge, and freezer

[*] http://www.parttimepaleobook.com

are going to be mostly vegetables, meat, fish, fowl, and eggs, with a few berries and miscellaneous fruits thrown in for good measure.

The rest of it is going to be the wonderful things you use to make the cooking magic happen—delicious things like coconut milk, butter/ghee, nuts, spices, butter . . . did I say butter twice? Butter is embraced in all but the most stringent Paleo crowds, and it's certainly on the yes list for anyone who's going Part-Time Paleo.

BETTER WITH BUTTER

Butter needs to be addressed as the exception to the Paleo no-dairy rule. It is, in essence, just another animal fat, but it's a special one with an incredible nutrient profile that isn't found elsewhere. As a matter of fact, the buzz in the nutrition world is that butter (the grass-fed variety) is beginning to emerge as the new superfood! Take that, cardiologists across the globe! That's right: Butter is better than just about anything else you might want to decorate your steamed veggies with.

Here's why butter is such a superstar:

- **CLA (conjugated linoleic acid).** This substance is known for its anti-inflammatory and anticancer properties.
- **Butyric acid (also known as butyrate).** This short-chain fatty acid has been shown to dramatically increase insulin sensitivity, is anti-inflammatory and anticancer, and helps control stress.
- **Beta-carotene.** A precursor to vitamin A, which is essential for the building of healthy skin, hair, and nails, beta-carotene helps to slow cognitive decline and is a top-notch scavenger of free radicals.
- **Vitamin K_2.** K_2 is the activator vitamin that has the ability to bind certain proteins that vitamins A and D produce. This means those same proteins will bind to the phosphorus and calcium found in your food and will be properly deposited in the bones and teeth instead of in the arteries (which would lead to atherosclerosis).

Let's celebrate butter by slathering it abundantly on our veggies tonight!

BASIC PALEO PANTRY STOCK-UP LIST

Now, remember, if it's perishable and not freezable the words *stock up* do not apply. But otherwise, keep as much of these items on hand as you have storage room for.

PANTRY

Nuts: walnuts, cashews, almonds, Brazil nuts, hazelnuts, pine nuts, macadamia nuts, pecans, pistachios . . . basically any nut but peanuts, because they are actually legumes

Seeds: pumpkin, sunflower, chia, sesame

Nut butters: almond, macadamia, sunflower

Honey: Make it local; keep it raw (mine is from my very own backyard bees!)

Dried fruit: raisins, currants, apricots, raw cacao nibs, unsweetened coconut flakes

Canned, jarred, or aseptic packed: tomatoes in any form, as long as you aren't sensitive to nightshades (sauce, crushed, diced, whole); chicken broth and beef broth (for emergencies only, because you'll be making your own!); anchovy paste; sardines; pumpkin; olives; coconut aminos; mustard; jarred ghee; canned coconut milk; aseptic-packed unsweetened coconut, almond, and hemp milks; coconut water; salsa; chipotle chilies (dried and in cans)

Teas: organic green, black, and white teas

Oils: walnut, macadamia nut, sesame, coconut, avocado

Vinegars: balsamic, rice, apple cider, red wine, white balsamic

Herbs and spices: basil, thyme, marjoram, oregano, nutmeg, peppercorns, sea salt, garlic and onion powders, curry powder, cayenne pepper, rosemary, sage, dill, fennel, cumin, coriander, cinnamon, bay leaves, ginger, herbs de Provence

Paleo-friendly flours and thickeners: coconut flour, almond flour, almond meal (almond meal is ground almonds with their skin on, and almond flour is made from blanched almonds with the skin removed), arrowroot flour, tapioca flour

Sea vegetables: dulse and kelp

Syrups: molasses, pure maple syrup

Treats: dark organic chocolate

COCONUT

Coconut Cream

There are so many delicious treats that nature has provided for us, and many of them have been forgotten with the introduction of processed foods and refined sugars.

Take coconut, for example. Coconuts are fatty, but the fat in our friend the coconut is used as a fuel source by our bodies when it's consumed, and it does not get stored in our butts or thighs.

Coconut Oil

Coconut oil is a miraculous product. It's a solid at room temperature, and when it warms up, it turns into a liquid. It is shelf stable in either form, and it can go from solid to liquid many times without its quality being jeopardized.

Use coconut oil to sauté with, to bake with, or even to moisturize your skin. There are hundreds of uses for coconut oil (just google it and you'll see what I'm talking about!), from softening dry lips to curing cradle cap.

Coconut oil can actually aid in weight loss because it burns stored fat in your body. It really is a miracle product. Look for organic, virgin (or unrefined) coconut oil, which is available in most mainstream grocery stores.

Bonus? It's delicious.

Coconut Butter

It's not really butter like we think of butter, but coconut butter (also referred to as coconut cream concentrate) is a concentrated form of coconut meat. The meat of the coconut is dried out and ground into a creamy consistency. Nothing is added to this delicious product (not even water), and it is absolutely delicious.

You can mix coconut butter with water to get coconut milk, put it in your coffee instead of cream, or use it in place of fruit dip or peanut butter. Oh so yummy! You'll find it in the health food section of most grocery stores. Or you can make your own coconut butter, simply by processing unsweetened coconut in your food processor or high-speed blender until it's smooth.

Coconut Milk

It's easier than ever before to get your hands on coconut milk. You can purchase two forms: carton or canned. I've personally replaced my cow's milk with coconut milk in the carton (So Delicious is a popular brand), and I use the canned stuff (richer, thicker, and higher in calories) in curry dishes and soups on a regular basis.

Coconut isn't just delicious; it's also full of nutrients. Your coconut "treat" will provide you with iron, vitamin C, copper, and manganese.

There is so much to love about coconuts. No wonder I'm crazy about 'em!

FRIDGE

Eggs: free-range organic

Milk: coconut and almond (both unsweetened)

Beverages: mineral water, green tea, filtered water, and mass quantities of wine

Condiments: mustard, sauerkraut, pickles, olives, horseradish, wasabi, Tabasco, Worcestershire (my favorite is the Wizard's organic), fish sauce (Red Boat brand)

Dairy: The only types of dairy you should have in your fridge must be organic—raw whole milk, plain Greek yogurt, kefir, and lots of grass-fed butter. Yes, I said raw whole milk. There are definitely safety concerns when it comes to consuming raw milk. But raw milk taken straight from the udder of a healthy, pastured cow should be perfectly safe . . . as long as it's handled and stored safely.

Ghee: butter that has undergone the simple process of clarification to remove the milk solids, leaving you with a glorious and nutritious golden liquid

Coffee: My absolute favorite is Bulletproof Coffee (see Resources).

FREEZER (OR FRIDGE IF YOU'RE GOING TO USE UP RIGHT AWAY)

Grass-fed beef: stew meat, short ribs, ground beef, roasts, steaks . . . any other cuts you like

Pastured pork: in any shape or form you want, including (hallelujah!) nitrate/nitrite-free bacon

Organic free-range chicken: whole and parts

Wild fish: Make sure it's not farm raised, ever, and do look for sustainable as well!

Bones: from pasture-raised, grass-fed chicken, beef, lamb, and pork; these gems are inexpensive and will become one of the healthiest things you can put in your body: bone broth (More later on this golden elixir and what to do with it.)

Berries: organic blueberries, raspberries, blackberries, strawberries, cherries, pomegranates, cranberries

Veggies: organic broccoli, green beans, pearl onions, leeks, bell pepper strips (unless you're sensitive to nightshades), cauliflower (you'll be eating a lot of it), spinach, dark leafy greens, kale, carrots, garlic, etc.

GHEE WHIZ!

Many of the recipes in this book call for ghee, which is a staple in the Part-Time Paleo kitchen.

Ghee, the beautiful golden liquid left behind when you remove the milk solids from butter, is a great dairy-free form of fat, and it is delicious.

You can buy ghee in well-stocked grocery stores, but it's dead easy to make your own. All you need to make ghee is some organic butter (preferably grass-fed) and a slow cooker.

Put eight sticks of butter in the slow cooker and leave it on low for about eight hours with something propping the lid open enough for steam to escape (a wooden spoon works).

Spoon the scum off the top of the two cups of liquid you're left with. Don't be tempted to scrape the sides and the bottom of the slow cooker to remove the burnt milk solids.

When the liquid comes to room temperature, filter it through cheesecloth and into a jar. You can store ghee in the fridge or in the cupboard.

WHERE TO SHOP

Now that you have a list, you're probably wondering where to get everything. I have some terrific resources for you online and offline and even some DIY ideas to help you keep costs in line.

Let's start with the stuff you can buy either at a farmers' market or through a CSA (community supported agriculture) program, in which you buy a "share" in the harvest and each week you receive your basket of goodies.

With a farmers' market, you need to remember only three things: 1) buy organic, 2) buy the freshest seasonal stuff available, and 3) go easy on the squash, sweet potatoes, etc. With a CSA basket, you get what you get. That's the advantage and disadvantage of a CSA—no choice.

That's not to say you can't get your produce at the grocery store. You certainly can. But keep this in mind: I strongly urge you to eat as organically as you possibly can, and you may not be able to do that 100 percent with the grocery store.

Going to a farmers' market for me is like going to Disneyland. It *is* the happiest place on earth. The gorgeous, locally grown produce lovingly just picked is absolute heaven. I buy whatever beautiful produce catches my eye, plus I get my eggs there, as well as my grass-fed beef and pork. Stocking up on local grass-fed meat is the most economical way to get bones for all those fabulous bone broths you'll be making.

While your first choice for food sources should be your local farmers' market or CSA, there is still a place in your shopping routine for big-box stores like Costco, BJ's, and their ilk. This is the place to pick up a lot of organic produce cheaply and to stock up on huge bags of organic carrots, onions, and celery.

You can also buy big tubs of organic baby spinach, spring mix for salads, and great blends of baby mixed greens (kale, chard, etc.) at those bulk food stores. Keep lots of greens on hand. I like to use the farmers' market greens for juicing; I will sauté the greens from BJ's as a side dish (with tons of garlic and ghee . . . yummy).

You'll want to buy your nuts, dried fruits, and Paleo flours in bulk because it's much more economical. You don't have to miss out on pancakes and pies just because you've adopted a new lifestyle (but go easy!). You just need to stock up on the necessary ingredients to make updated versions of your family's favorites.

BACKYARD ANIMAL HUSBANDRY

While it might not be feasible to keep a cow in your backyard (the HOA is likely to get wind—literally and figuratively—of an eight-hundred-pound animal helping you keep the grass trimmed), chickens are another matter entirely.

Chicken keeping has been growing in popularity across North America. Williams-Sonoma even has cute chicken coops for sale on their website (if you don't mind shelling out about a thousand bucks).

As one who has been there, done that with the whole chicken thing, I can tell you it does take a little work, but the eggs are well worth the small effort you put out daily to keep your hens happy.

Farm-fresh free-range eggs are a critical aspect of Paleo eating. That's because the eggs of free-range chickens are much more nutritious than those of factory-farmed chickens. Factory-farmed chickens are usually fed grains and soy, whereas free-range chickens eat bugs and grass, like chickens should.

DIY PALEO CONDIMENTS

Once you go even the tiniest bit Paleo, you'll discover those familiar condiments that were once staples of your grocery list are now off-limits. Just take a gander at that ketchup label and check out the list of obnoxious ingredients. Betcha didn't know there was corn syrup or worse, high-fructose corn syrup, lurking in there, did you?

The mayo has to go, too, since it's usually made from evil GMO canola or soy oil. The salad dressings? Forget it. They're chock-full of nasty oils, chemicals, and preservatives, too.

The good news for you is that it's easy to make your own condiments as you need them. Really, there's nothing to it.

Homemade Paleo Ketchup

All you need to make your own ketchup is tomatoes, some vinegar, something sweet (I like honey), and some spices. Experiment with recipes until you find one that your family enjoys. My go-to is a can of organic tomato paste with a dollop of honey, some organic apple cider vinegar, a pinch of both onion powder and garlic powder, a pinch of allspice, and some salt and pepper. Add a little bit of water and bring to a boil. Simmer until it looks like ketchup!

Homemade Paleo Mustard

Making mustard is even easier than making ketchup. Mix a half cup of mustard powder with a half cup of water and a pinch of sea salt. You're done.

Homemade Paleo Mayo

Home chefs everywhere are intimidated by the thought of making mayonnaise. And it can be tricky. If you get a little too eager with adding the oil, your mayo can break. If you take your time and use the best ingredients you can, you'll be just fine.

For starters, I recommend using a stick blender for making mayo, but you can use a whisk or a food processor. To make about one cup of mayo, you'll need one cold egg, one room temperature lemon, a pinch of mustard powder, and a half cup of lightly colored oil. You can use light olive oil, avocado oil, or macadamia oil—whichever light oil you like best.

Crack your egg into a bowl; add the juice of half a lemon and your mustard powder. Start to blend with your immersion blender and begin adding your oil, a few drops at a time, until your mayo starts to thicken. As you get closer to the consistency of mayo, you can add your oil in a steadier stream. When it looks like it's done, stop! It doesn't take much to break your mayo, taking it from thick and creamy to watery and unusable! It will last for about a week in the fridge.

Homemade Paleo Tomato Dill Relish

The purpose of relish is to enhance a meal. We're mostly familiar with hot dog relish, but relish can be anything you want it to be. Mix up some diced cucumber and fresh dill with your favorite vinegar, some lemon juice, olive oil, and salt and pepper, and just add stuff until you get a taste you love. This tomato dill relish is wonderful with fish:

2 cups diced roma (plum) tomatoes
½ cup diced red onion
½ cup diced cucumber
¼ cup finely chopped dill
2 tablespoons balsamic vinegar
3 tablespoons lemon juice
3 tablespoons extra virgin olive oil
Sea salt and freshly ground black pepper to taste

Homemade Paleo Salsa

Making your own salsa is as easy as chopping vegetables. You may have to chop until you drop, but the fresh flavor will be worth it.

Your basic ingredients will be roma tomatoes, onions, bell peppers, jalapeños, lime juice, salt, and cilantro. Taste-test until you get it just right. Once you have the basic formula down, have fun with it. Separate your salsa into little batches, to which you can add all kinds of things. Add in some avocado, mango, strawberries, pineapple, black beans . . . you're limited only by your imagination!

As a bonus, salsa freezes really well. Freeze it in very small batches, so you can thaw out enough for one meal at a time.

Now that you know what items you'll want to be stocking up on, it's time to take a closer look at how and why you're going to be eating this stuff.

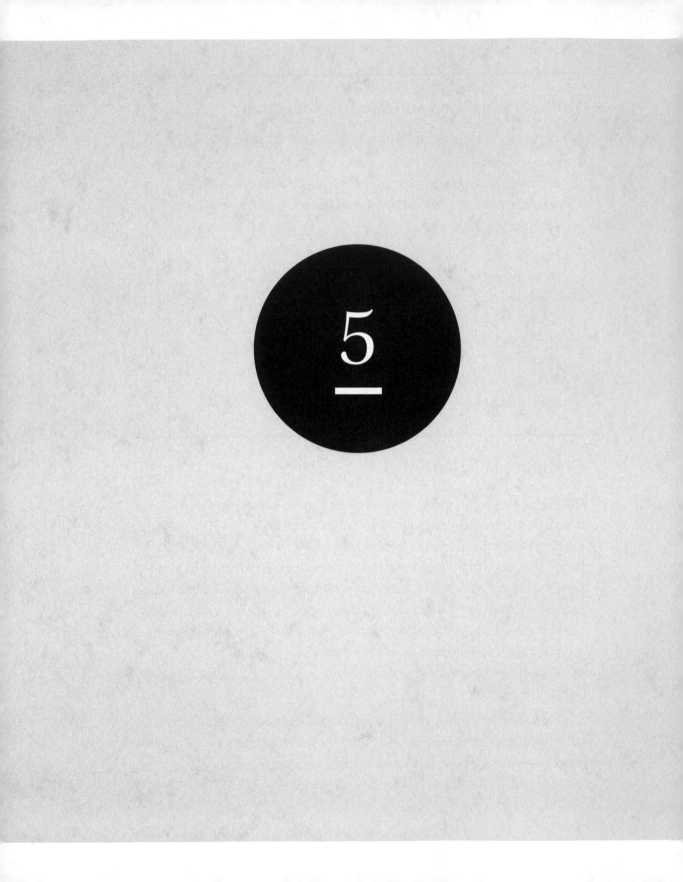

CHAPTER FIVE

PRODUCE AND PALEO

T here's a bit of a misconception out there that when you're Paleo, you eat pounds and pounds of meat each day. But that's not entirely true. Yes, we eat meat, but we go heavy on the veggies, too. In fact, believe it or not, true vegans and Paleoistas are not that far off from each other. The difference is vegans eat grains, legumes, and beans, and we eat animal products. Vegans and Paleo eaters both know that mighty nutrient-dense plants need to make up the bulk of the diet.

That's probably contrary to what a lot of people think about eating a Paleo-based diet. I've been asked many, many times, "What's the difference between eating Paleo and Atkins?" These are sincere people asking sincere questions, because Paleo is often confused with eating great portions of meat, eggs, and bacon.

Yes, there's meat involved in eating the way our ancestors ate, but we need to remember that they weren't just hunters. They were also gatherers, and the "gathering" portion of eating was more prevalent than the eating-after-the-hunt portion. Primitive societies were consummate "avail-avarians." That is, they ate what was readily available. It was somewhat imbalanced at times—they might gorge themselves after a big kill on a lot of protein, then not have any for a week or more, eating only the vegetation they could find or dig up.

SQUARE FOOT GARDENING

There really aren't any excuses for not growing your own food. It doesn't matter where you live or how green your thumb is; you can manage a two-foot-by-four-foot garden.

Square foot gardening is enjoying popularity now with the surging local-food movement. City dwellers with no yards to speak of are planting food in tiny plots of earth. Busy working parents in rural settings who don't have time to tend to a large garden patch are harvesting beautiful organic veggies from small and manageable square foot spaces.

To get started with your own square foot garden, pick a location that will get at least six to eight hours of direct sun per day. Ideally, the space will be away from trees and shrubs so that shadows and roots don't interfere with your planting. Then, build or buy a box frame six inches high—only large enough for you to maintain. Lay down some cardboard, and then top the box up with a combination of soil, compost, vermiculite, and peat moss. Create a foot-by-foot grid pattern and then start planting.

One of the great things about square foot gardening is that you hardly get any weeds. The layer of cardboard (even newspaper would work) on the bottom of the box will help to prevent pesky weeds from poking through. And the raised sides of the box will help keep them from creeping in from the sides.

You can google this to death. There is a ton of information out there about square foot gardening. So, go on and get your hands dirty. It is so unbelievably rewarding to harvest a feed of ripe tomatoes and bright green kale from your very own yard. You are going to love it.

I'm not one of those who romanticize our ancestors' "perfect" diet. They had their nutritional struggles like we do, although they weren't because of fast food and Doritos. The difference was they listened to their bodies and would seek out the nutrients they needed, often traveling great distances to get that particular food.

The biggest needle mover, in my opinion, for making a significant change in your health is getting the micronutrients into your body via a whole lot of veggies. This is a significant part of a truly nutrient-rich Paleo diet and one that cannot be overlooked.

Terry Wahls, MD, is an important mentor and friend of mine. Her viral video about her journey of healing herself from progressive secondary multiple sclerosis through diet changed my whole view of nutrition in about eighteen minutes. I've always been a firm believer in eating healthy, organic whole foods and have been speaking passionately about this subject to anyone who'd listen for more than twenty years. But this woman's impassioned TED talk about getting out of her wheelchair and taking an eighteen-mile bike trek within that same year made me totally reassess the importance of food and, specifically, the Paleo diet.

The key to the Paleo lifestyle is eating organic produce as much as possible. Our hunter-gatherer ancestors didn't have to tiptoe around Monsanto in the wild. The introduction of chemicals into our food chain is a major problem, and it is important to eat organic over conventionally grown produce.

But for those of us without an unlimited food budget, we need to be realistic. It is more important to get eight or nine cups of produce into you per day (yes, you need that many!) than to worry about each and every one of those veggies being organic. But there are some foods that are the exception to this, because they are generally sprayed quite heavily with pesticides.

THE DIRTY DOZEN

To help you decide what you should buy organic and what you can skimp on a bit, the Dirty Dozen (which the Environmental Working Group* updates every year) lists the twelve foods that should be avoided altogether if organic is not available, because of the high amounts of pesticides found on or in them. Because this list changes annually, you will want to make sure the following is still accurate at the time you're reading this!

---

* ewg.org

- **Apples.** That nonorganic apple could have up to forty different pesticides on it. That's because insects and fungus love apples even more than we do, and so farmers are forced to spray the heck out of their orchards. This means that apple juice and applesauce can also be heavy on pesticides if you don't choose organic options. If organic apples aren't available, at the very least discard the peels. Keep in mind, though, that when you do that, you lose most of the nutrients of the fruit.
- **Celery.** Up to sixty different pesticides have been detected on nonorganic celery. If you can't find it organic, you should look for your crunch elsewhere.
- **Strawberries.** Strawberries are lousy with chemicals and pesticide residue because, just as with apples, bugs love them. If you don't have an organic strawberry option, consider reaching for a different type of berry.
- **Peaches.** Farmers use up to sixty different chemicals to rid their peach trees of pests. For that reason, avoid peaches that are not organic. This goes for canned peaches as well.
- **Spinach.** The leafy green with the highest amount of pesticides is spinach. This goes for the frozen variety, too, by the way. Buy it organic, or buy a different green leafy veggie.
- **Imported nectarines.** Did you know that imported nectarines are among the most contaminated tree fruits out there? Though they're not as bad, domestic nectarines are still high in pesticide residue, so if you can't find organic, buy something else.
- **Grapes.** Grapes are a filthy food item, with more than thirty pesticides being used to grow them. Buy organic grapes and raisins, and look for organic wine.
- **Sweet bell peppers.** No matter what color you reach for, your sweet bell peppers are covered in pesticide residue if they're not organic.
- **Potatoes.** Potatoes are so high in pesticides that potato farmers won't even eat them! Sweet potatoes are more nutritious and have less pesticide residue than their white relatives, so buy those if you can't find organic spuds. (And we want to avoid white potatoes anyway!)

- **Cucumbers.** These are a favorite of mine, especially for juicing. Not only important due to pesticide residues, but conventional cucumbers are waxed—yuck.
- **Imported snap peas.** Perfect for stir fries, the sweet crunch of snap peas are also great in salads and as a side dish, but be sure to get organic snap peas. If they're not available, make sure they are at least grown stateside.
- **Cherry tomatoes.** New to the Dirty Dozen list, cherry tomatoes are a staple in many people's fridge (mine included) for salads, snacking, and a nice punch of color to incorporate into side dishes. Make sure they're organic though!

THE CLEAN 15

Now that we know which foods are dirtiest, let's look at the Clean 15! These are vegetables that are generally safe to eat in a nonorganic form. I still advise that you look for organic when possible (with the exception of avocados and bananas, because of their thick skins) and to always wash your fruits and veggies.

- Onions
- Avocados
- Corn*
- Pineapples
- Mango
- Asparagus
- Sweet peas
- Cabbage
- Kiwi

---

* As you will read later, corn is generally not a good food to eat, and honestly, I don't feel that it should be included in this list. But this isn't my list; it's from ewg.org.

- Eggplant
- Cantaloupe
- Papaya
- Grapefruit
- Cauliflower
- Sweet potatoes

PALEO JUICE

Modern living is nutrient depleting in many ways. To start with, our produce isn't as rich in nutrients as it once was, thanks to the deteriorating quality of soil, pesticides, chemicals, and GMOs.

In addition to these nutritionally inferior fruits and vegetables, modern humans tend to eat refined sugars, alcohol, and caffeine. If you smoke, there are more chemicals to worry about. (Stop smoking!) These little habits damage a lot of that nutrient-rich food and those vitamin supplements before you have a chance to absorb it.

Because of all the damage the Standard American Diet does to the human digestive system, most of us have at least a small degree of gut damage that is affecting our digestion. If your digestion isn't optimal, you might be losing up to half of the nutrients you do take in due to poor absorption.

Juicing every day can help you get a boost of nutrition straight to your cells. Drinking pure juice is an efficient way to deliver nutrient-rich and highly absorbable vegetables into your bloodstream. It flushes out chemicals and toxins and makes you feel amazing.

But I'm not talking about juicing berries and fruit here. This juice needs to be green so that you can avoid unnecessary carbs and sugars.

You will want to focus on veggies like kale, parsley, tomatoes, carrots, spinach, Swiss chard, celery, cucumbers, and beets. It's okay to use a green apple in there (just a half) to sweeten the juice once in a while, but don't go crazy.

The best way to juice kale, chard, and parsley is to roll them into a tight bundle and force it through the juicer with a carrot or a different firm veggie.

As a general rule, drink one big serving of green juice per day. You can find good, inexpensive juicers or splurge for a high-speed Blendtec blender. (You will have to strain the juice from the pulp with your blender, but a juicer does that step for you.)

If you can't stand tossing out the fiber from the juice of those fruits and veggies, save it—or at least some of it. Put it in soups or a pot of chili. I find it's helpful to freeze my juice pulp in portions so that I have roughage to toss into my bone broths and stocks. Then I get all the good out of those pricey organic foods!

Eating the right foods isn't just about fitting into your skinny jeans and looking good. Hippocrates got it right so many centuries ago: "Natural forces within us are the true healers of disease."

That means we need to eat the right foods to fuel those "natural forces," as Hippocrates so eloquently put it. You can't run a car on just any strong-smelling liquid, any more than you can enjoy good health if you eat any solid that claims to be "food." It takes the right fuels for both bodies and cars to run, and it takes great fuel for both to run optimally.

The starting place for this optimal fuel begins with micronutrient-dense fruits and vegetables (but mostly vegetables).

EAT YOUR VEGGIES

Here are my top five ways to get those veggies in:

1. **Juice.** Green juices are an amazing way to get your veggie quota up each day. I drink one glass of fresh juice every single day, typically kale (or another powerhouse green), celery, cucumber, parsley, carrot, and maybe half a green apple. All ingredients are, of course, organic.

2. **Soup.** My Mighty Mitochondria Soup is made of bone broth and every veggie you need to get your nutrient quota up. Having a cup before lunch and/or dinner will boost your nutrients.

3. **Salad.** A big salad (I do two handfuls for my side salad, each day for each meal) is just the ticket. From there, you can add a plethora of fixings and really knock it out of the park nutrient-wise.

4. **Green smoothies.** Sometimes I get burned out on juicing or I just get lazy. Juicing is more work than making a smoothie. That's because you have to strain the pulp from the Blendtec to get the juice, or you have to go to the trouble of cleaning the juicer. With a smoothie, you just toss everything in the blender and drink the whole works. You can also add some good healthy fat and protein to a smoothie, which you can't do with juicing. I add a handful or two of organic baby spinach to my morning smoothie. If you have blueberries in there and a great-tasting protein powder, you don't even notice!

5. **Sprouts.** I keep sprouts going on my countertop. I add these power-houses to my salads each day. I also tend to grab a handful of them and munch while I'm making my juice. It sounds hard-core, I know (and maybe it is?), but I know how these little tiny superfoods make me feel: awesome!

SPROUTING OFF

There are 101 reasons why you should eat sprouts. One of the biggest is that they are incredible superfoods with very little cost. But here are four more reasons why you need sprouts in your life:

• **Oxygen rich.** Raw foods contain oxygen, and cooking those foods destroys that oxygen. Did you know that cancer cells can't live in oxygen-rich environments? Sprouts are full of oxygen, and eating them raw on a regular basis is very good for us.

- **Alkaline rich.** Sprouts have an alkaline effect on our bodies. Our immune systems are strengthened by alkalizing foods like sprouts. Cancer cells also can't thrive in an alkaline-rich environment.
- **Antioxidant rich.** Sprouts from radish, broccoli, clover, and alfalfa are abundant in disease-fighting compounds called phytochemicals. They're also rich in antioxidants, which protect against disease.
- **Nutrient rich.** Sprouts have more nutrients in them than fully mature plants do. Think about it: The sprout contains the nutrition it needs to get the plant to grow. For example, a cup of raw or cooked broccoli contains 1.5 milligrams of vitamin E, while a cup of broccoli sprouts contains 7.5 mg. That cup of cooked broccoli contains 1.5 mg of selenium, while its sprouted equivalent has up to 28 mg. Now, you aren't likely to sit down with a cup of broccoli sprouts, but that should give you an idea of just how nutritious these little guys are.

Not only are they healthy, but sprouts are delicious, too. I sprout my own radish (spicy!) and broccoli seeds and eat them in salads nearly every day. I'm fond of alfalfa sprouts as well.

I highly recommend that you grow your own sprouts. Those sprouts in the stores are not only expensive, but they have also been known to contain salmonella and mold. Yuck!

How to Grow Your Own Sprouts

When you sprout your own seeds, you'll have delicious additions to your meals within a few days. The jar method is as easy as pie. All you need are some organic sprouting seeds or beans (buy them at your local health food store or online), wide-mouth mason jars, and sprouting lids for the jars. If you can't find the lids, you can use rubber bands and cheesecloth.

1. After washing your hands, remove any discolored or broken seeds before placing a tablespoon of seeds or a third of a cup of beans (mung bean sprouts are wonderful and they're the kind we're generally most familiar with) or grains (try barley, rye, or wheat) into the jar. (Once grains are sprouted, they are now plants, and therefore fair game to consume!) Cover those seeds or beans with pure water. (Use a cup to cover a tablespoon of seeds or one-third cup of beans, nuts, or grains.) Use a different jar for each type of sprouts and you'll have a nice variety to choose from.

2. Let the seeds or beans soak for six to twelve hours. (I just let them soak overnight.) After they've soaked, cover the jar with cheesecloth and a rubber band or with a sprouting lid and then drain off the water.

3. After draining, rinse the beans or seeds with fresh water and drain again. Place the jar on its side in a cool, clean spot in the kitchen. Place something under the bottom of the bottle so it's propped up at a slight angle, allowing any excess water to drain off of the beans or the seeds.

4. A few times a day, give them a good rinse and drain them very well. Keep the jar tilted down. Within a few days you'll have a jar full of gorgeous little sprouts.

How's that for easy?

The biggest push-back I get from people trying this lifestyle is the cost of the fresh produce. And I won't deny that fresh, organic produce isn't cheap. But I would much rather spend my money now on health-promoting foods than spend it later on medicine and hospital stays.

HOW TO GROW YOUR LETTUCE (NO MATTER WHERE YOU LIVE!)

It can get expensive eating the amount of greens that you need. That's why I was thrilled to find a lettuce bowl at my local nursery. I immediately brought it home and then figured out how to do it myself so I can teach you all about it!

Here's what you'll need:

- A large round planting pot, about six inches deep (or a BPA-free container of some sort with roughly the same depth)
- Some organic potting soil (Look for the kind with perlite in it—that's those little round white balls you see in the dirt mixture)
- Mesclun mix seeds (or whatever lettuce you like best)
- Water (I know, duh!)
- A sunny window (It should get at least six hours of sun a day. Not enough sun makes lettuce tall and lanky, not bushy and wonderful.)

To make your lettuce bowl:

1. Fill your container to the halfway mark with soil. You can sprinkle some fertilizer on there if you want to. Moisten the soil and sprinkle a couple of pinches of seeds on top. Sprinkle a little more soil over the seeds and spritz the surface with more water.
2. Water daily and keep the pot in the sun or under a grow light. The seeds should sprout up in about seven days and your first harvest should be ready in about a month—yay!

Super easy, right?

To harvest your lettuce:

After you cut your lettuce the first time (leave those growing crowns that you snip the lettuce from alone!), you'll only have to wait another two weeks for a fresh crop.

But here's an idea to keep the lettuce going: Get another lettuce bowl started a week after the first one so you have a harvest every week! Ta-da!

Instead of griping about the cost of fresh produce, I think we should normalize the great value these amazing foods hold. They feed your body, nourishing every cell you have and giving your mitochondria the fuel they need to do their job; there really is no substitute. You cannot feed your body in any other way and still have good health. This is huge.

The fact is we are willing to give Starbucks five dollars a day for a fancy, sugary, health-robbing coffee that we don't need instead of spending that same amount of money on organic produce that we require. Yes, *require*. You cannot argue with physiology. Our bodies cannot adapt to cheap junk food; they just get sick. Once we realize that everything that goes in our mouths will either promote or destroy our health, the choices become a lot easier to make.

Unfortunately, it's not enough to just say, "Eat your vegetables." You can't have one salad and think you've covered your bases for the day. The fact is we need a wide variety of veggies. The starting point is with lots of leafy greens, such as various lettuces, spinach, and chard, as well as lesser-known and underused greens like dandelion greens, turnip greens, beet greens, and watercress, to name a few.

Greens are heavy on the B vitamins, which are important for the brain to operate optimally. These are the vitamins that control mood, focus, learning, and impulse control. Leafy greens also contain a fair amount of beta-carotene, a precursor to vitamin A, which helps build healthy skin, muscles, and hair. Beta-carotene may also protect your skin against sun damage.

Other antioxidants found in greens include vitamins C and E, as well as lutein and zeaxanthin—important nutrients that help prevent macular degeneration and may even help improve vision.

We also need sulfur-containing vegetables such as cauliflower, broccoli, cabbage, kale, collard greens, onions, leeks, and garlic. You know sulfury-smelling veggies, right? Except for the onions, leeks, and garlic, when you cook any other sulfur-rich veggie, you end up with a very distinct smell—that's the sulfur compounds making their way into your olfactory system.

Dr. Wahls gets the credit for helping me (and millions of others) understand the importance of eating a wide variety of vegetables. They each have specific characteristics, and sulfur-containing veggies are some of the most potent anticancer foods on the planet. Add the antioxidant component and the liver protection offered by these sulfurous friends and you've got yourself some powerhouse foods.

Next up is eating your colors. If you can focus on making a colorful dish when you build a salad or place veggies on your plate, then eating healthfully becomes simple.

I believe we crave beauty naturally, and a beautiful plate of food is no different. If it is all white (chicken breast, cauliflower, and spaghetti squash on a white plate, for example), we will naturally recoil and say, "Eww, that looks awful." However, if we see a steak piled with mushrooms and onions, served with some baked sweet potatoes and steamed broccoli, we'll say, "Yum, that looks delicious!" One plate is bland and uninviting; the other is colorful and gorgeous and makes you want to dig right in!

So back to the colors we need to eat. Those phytonutrient-rich peppers, carrots, and tomatoes are a pleasure to look at as well as eat. Choosing a variety of colors in your food will help you cover your nutrient needs and pleasure your palate as well.

CORN-FUSED ABOUT CORN?

Most people are, because it's not what you think it is. The fact is, corn isn't a vegetable—it's a grain! That takes it off our Paleo plates, then, doesn't it? But there's more you need to know about corn.

Most corn in North America is grown from genetically modified seed. The seeds themselves contain pesticides so that insects die when they eat the crop. Do some research on GMO if this is a new concept for you, and you'll quickly see why this is such a big deal. But that's another book for another day!

Besides the GMO factor, corn is at the top of the glycemic index because it's teeming with sugar. Did you know a piece of cornbread has a higher glycemic index than a piece of pound cake? More than double!

Corn shows up in most processed foods, from corn syrup to corn oil to hydrogenated vegetable oils, which are some of the most potent anti-nutrients on the planet. So it's not just corn on the cob or frozen and canned corn you have to beware of. Do yourself a favor and skip corn in all of its evil forms by diligently reading your labels.

FRUIT

So what about fruit on the Part-Time Paleo plan? I am so glad you asked! The best fruits are colored all the way through from skin to interior, indicating a higher nutrient value than fruits that are colorful on the outside but not on the inside. Berries are the optimal expression of good fruit choices. They are full of fiber and low in sugar, and most can be classified as a superfood for all the good they do in our bodies.

Berries (all of them, by the way) are prime-time antioxidant superstars, filled to the brim with polyphenols that cool off inflammation and may even relieve pain due to their salicylic acid content.

I keep a wide variety of organic berries in my freezer and change them out in my daily smoothie so I get a full range of health benefits with the different types. I also find the flavor and variety keeps me from getting bored.

Besides berries, I also love cherries. They are extremely flavorful and, once again, they follow the color rule (deeply hued all the way through). Did you know that cherries can actually help relieve gout pain by about 35 percent, according to a Boston University study? This is most likely due to the cherry's amazing anti-inflammatory properties, such as vitamin C and anthocyanins—the water-soluble plant pigments that work miracles in our bodies.

Avocados, apricots, grapefruit, oranges, lemons, limes, grapes, plums, pomegranates, rhubarb, and kiwi are solid-colored fruits that are mostly lower on the glycemic index. I don't know about you, but I can go crazy eating summer fruits, so just keep in mind that while they all have loads of nutrition, they also have loads of sugar. Yes, it's natural sugar, but it will also "naturally" put the weight on you and around your belly unless you practice the moderation rule.

MAKE YOUR OWN SALAD BAR

Salads are a major part of any Paleo diet. A great way to simplify salad making is to create your own salad bar. This is one of my tricks for getting a nutritious salad done quickly. I use a multitude of containers with prepped veggies stacked in my produce bin—all the time.

This is how it's done:

- **Containers.** Ideally, you need squarish or rectangular containers to avoid wasted space in your produce bin. I use Rubbermaid, which has differing sizes that work well.

- **Veggie prep.** You will need to prep your veggies all at once. Shred your carrots, chop some onion, slice some cukes, and wash some grape tomatoes for the containers.
- **Replenish when finished.** Make sure you use up what's in each container before adding more. This will keep your prepped produce fresher and better.

All you need to do to whip up a quick and healthy salad for lunch or dinner is put a couple of big handfuls of greens in a bowl and top it however you like. A great way to put some color on your plate without having to take too much time to chop is to make ribbons of carrot with a plain old veggie peeler. Your dressing needn't be any more complicated than a mixture of quality extra virgin olive oil and a good vinegar.

JUICING

Now that you know what fruits and veggies are the most critical to purchase in their organic form, it's time to start juicing!

The following juice and smoothie recipes will make it a cinch for you to get in a ton of those important micronutrients.

PART-TIME PALEO JUICE AND SMOOTHIE RECIPES

Super Green Juice

Yields 1 serving

2 carrots
½ green apple

½ orange, peeled, leaving pith

½ lemon, peeled, leaving pith

1 slice ginger, ¼ inch thick

1 red chard leaf

1 cup fresh parsley

5 kale leaves

½ cup arugula

Wash and dry all ingredients, and run through the juicer one at a time. For small leaves, like parsley, bunch them together tightly to form a "solid" leaf vegetable for better juicing. Chill with ice (if desired; it's always best to drink it right away), stir, and enjoy.

Strawberry Basil Juice with a Twist

Yields 1 serving

½ cup strawberries

4 large celery stalks

2 turnips

½ cup basil

½ cup parsley

½ carrot

¼ lemon, peeled, leaving pith

1 cup spinach

5 kale leaves

Wash and dry all ingredients, and run through the juicer one at a time. For smaller leaves, like basil and parsley, bunch them together tightly to form a "solid" leaf vegetable for better juicing. Chill (if desired), stir, and enjoy.

Mango Carrot Juice

Yields 1 serving

- ½ cup mango, pitted, not peeled
- 5 carrots
- 1 cup spinach
- ¼ orange, peeled, leaving pith
- 10 kale leaves
- 1 stalk celery

Wash and dry all ingredients, and run through the juicer one at a time. Chill (if desired), stir, and enjoy.

Hawaiian Island Juice

Yields 1 serving

- ½ coconut, use the flesh and reserve coconut water for a smoothie (or something else)
- 2 carrots
- ½ cup pineapple
- 1 cup spinach
- 2 stalks celery
- 5 kale leaves
- ½ lime, peeled, leaving pith
- ¼ orange, peeled, leaving pith
- 1 slice ginger, ¼ inch thick
- ½ cucumber

Wash and dry all ingredients, and run through the juicer one at a time, starting with the coconut. Follow immediately with the carrots to avoid the coconut getting "stuck." Chill (if desired), stir, and enjoy.

Spicy Tango Salsa Juice

Yields 1 serving

  1 green apple
  1 peach, pitted, not peeled
  ½ clove garlic
  2 tomatoes
  ½ jalapeño
  ½ lime, peeled, leaving pith
  1 cup spinach
  ¼ cup cilantro
  5 kale leaves
  ¼ red onion

Wash and dry all ingredients, and run through the juicer one at a time. Run the ingredients through in the order listed to be sure you get the maximum juice from smaller ingredients (i.e., garlic, jalapeño). For smaller leaves, like cilantro, bunch them together tightly to form a "solid" leaf vegetable for better juicing. Chill (if desired), stir, and enjoy.

Apple Spiced Juice

Yields 1 serving

  2 apples
  ½ orange, peeled, leaving pith
  1 cup spinach
  5 kale leaves
  ½ cup parsley
  1 pinch Ceylon cinnamon (optional)

Wash and dry all ingredients, and run through the juicer one at a time, except the cinnamon. For smaller leaves, like parsley, bunch them together tightly to form a "solid" leaf vegetable for better juicing. Chill (if desired), stir in cinnamon (if desired), and enjoy.

Honeyloupe Garden Juice

Yields 1 serving

¼ cantaloupe, peeled and seeded
¼ honeydew, peeled and seeded
½ grapefruit
2 tomatoes
½ cup spinach
½ fennel bulb
1 carrot
3 kale leaves
½ cup parsley

Wash and dry all ingredients, and run through the juicer one at a time. For smaller leaves, like parsley, bunch them together tightly to form a "solid" leaf vegetable for better juicing. Chill (if desired), stir, and enjoy.

Green Beet Juice

Yields 1 serving

2 beets
2 carrots
1 slice ginger, ¼ inch thick
½ lime, peeled, leaving pith
½ cucumber
1 cup spinach
5 kale leaves
½ cup parsley

Wash and dry all ingredients, and run through the juicer one at a time. For smaller leaves, like parsley, bunch them together tightly to form a "solid" leaf vegetable for better juicing. Chill (if desired), stir, and enjoy.

Dandelion Citrus Juice

Yields 1 serving

- 1 cup dandelion greens
- 1 orange, peeled, leaving pith
- ½ lemon, peeled, leaving pith
- ½ lime, peeled, leaving pith
- 1 slice ginger, ¼ inch thick
- 1 cup spinach
- 5 kale leaves
- ½ chard leaf
- 1 cup parsley

Wash and dry all ingredients, and run through the juicer one at a time. For smaller leaves, like parsley, bunch them together tightly to form a "solid" leaf vegetable for better juicing. Chill (if desired), stir, and enjoy.

Apple, Apricot, Dandelion, Kale, and Spinach Juice

Yields 1 serving

- 1 cup dandelion greens
- 2 apples
- 1 apricot, pitted
- 1 thick slice bitter melon
- 1 slice ginger, ¼ inch thick
- 1 cup spinach
- 5 kale leaves

2 stalks celery

1 cup parsley

Wash and dry all ingredients, and run through the juicer one at a time. For smaller leaves, like parsley, bunch them together tightly to form a "solid" leaf vegetable for better juicing. Chill (if desired), stir, and enjoy.

Raspberry Cobbler Smoothie

Yields 1 serving

¼ cup coconut cream

¼ cup unsweetened almond milk, or use a different Paleo-friendly milk

1 banana

½ cup frozen raspberries

1 scoop All-in-One Vanilla Smoothie Mix (see Resources)

1 scoop FiberMender (see Resources)

Place coconut cream, almond milk, and banana in blender. Blend until combined. Add raspberries, Smoothie Mix, and FiberMender. Blend until smooth and enjoy.

Green Berry Smoothie

Yields 1 serving

½ cup unsweetened coconut milk, like So Delicious, or use a different milk

¼ cup frozen mixed berries

½ cup spinach

2 tablespoons honey

1 scoop All-in-One Vanilla Smoothie Mix (see Resources)

1 scoop FiberMender (see Resources)

Place coconut milk, then mixed berries and spinach in blender. Blend until combined. Add honey, Smoothie Mix, and FiberMender. Blend until smooth and enjoy.

Blue/Cran Berry Smoothie

Yields 1 serving

   ¼ cup unsweetened almond milk, or use a different milk

   ¼ cup unsweetened 100 percent cranberry juice

   ½ cup frozen blueberries

   2 teaspoons palm sugar or a pinch of stevia

   1 scoop All-in-One Vanilla Smoothie Mix (see Resources)

   1 scoop FiberMender (see Resources)

Place almond milk, cranberry juice, and blueberries in blender. Blend until mostly combined. Add sugar or stevia, Smoothie Mix, and FiberMender. Blend until smooth and enjoy.

Tropical Basil Smoothie

Yields 1 serving

   ¼ cup unsweetened coconut milk, like So Delicious, or use a different milk

   2 tablespoons unsweetened almond milk, or use a different milk

   ¼ orange, peeled, leaving pith

   ½ cup frozen pineapple

   ¼ teaspoon coconut extract

   2 tablespoons honey

   ¼ cup basil

   1 scoop All-in-One Vanilla Smoothie Mix (see Resources)

   1 scoop FiberMender (see Resources)

Place coconut milk, almond milk, orange, pineapple, and coconut extract in blender. Blend until mostly combined. Add honey, basil, Smoothie Mix, and FiberMender. Blend until smooth and enjoy.

Almond Cherry Bliss Smoothie

Yields 1 serving

¼ cup unsweetened almond milk, or use a different milk

¼ cup 100 percent cranberry juice

½ cup frozen, pitted cherries

¼ teaspoon almond extract

2 teaspoons palm sugar or a pinch of stevia

1 scoop All-in-One Vanilla Smoothie Mix (see Resources)

1 scoop FiberMender (see Resources)

Place almond milk, cranberry juice, cherries, and almond extract in blender. Blend until mostly combined. Add palm sugar or stevia, Smoothie Mix, and FiberMender. Blend until smooth and enjoy.

Coconut Green Smoothie

Yields 1 serving

⅓ cup unsweetened coconut milk, like So Delicious, or use a different milk

⅓ cup crushed ice

¼ cup spinach

¼ cup kale

¼ cup green apple

1 teaspoon honey

1 scoop All-in-One Vanilla Smoothie Mix (see Resources)

1 scoop FiberMender (see Resources)

Place coconut milk and crushed ice in blender. Blend until mostly combined. Add spinach, kale, apple, honey, Smoothie Mix, and FiberMender. Blend until smooth and enjoy. This is a thick smoothie. It's okay to add a tad more milk of your choice, if a thinner texture is preferred.

Avocado Kale Smoothie

Yields 1 serving

⅓ cup unsweetened coconut milk, like So Delicious, or use a different milk
⅓ cup crushed ice
¼ cup kale
2 kiwi, peeled
½ avocado
1 teaspoon palm sugar or a pinch of stevia
1 scoop All-in-One Vanilla Smoothie Mix (see Resources)
1 scoop FiberMender (see Resources)

Place coconut milk and crushed ice in blender. Blend until mostly combined. Add kale, kiwi, avocado, palm sugar or stevia, Smoothie Mix, and FiberMender. Blend until smooth and enjoy. This is a thick smoothie. It's okay to add a tad more milk of your choice, if a thinner texture is preferred.

Strawberry Spinach Salad Smoothie

Yields 1 serving

¼ cup unsweetened coconut milk, like So Delicious, or use a different milk
¼ cup 100 percent cranberry juice
¼ cup spinach
¼ cup frozen strawberries
1 teaspoon honey
1 scoop All-in-One Vanilla Smoothie Mix (see Resources)
1 scoop FiberMender (see Resources)

Place coconut milk, cranberry juice, spinach, and strawberries in blender. Blend until mostly combined. Add honey, Smoothie Mix, and FiberMender. Blend until smooth and enjoy.

Apricot Berry Smoothie

Yields 1 serving

- ¼ cup unsweetened coconut milk, like So Delicious, or use a different milk
- ¼ cup 100 percent cranberry juice
- ½ cup frozen or fresh apricots, pitted
- 1 teaspoon palm sugar or a pinch of stevia
- 1 scoop All-in-One Vanilla Smoothie Mix (see Resources)
- 1 scoop FiberMender (see Resources)

Place coconut milk, cranberry juice, and apricots in blender. Blend until mostly combined. Add palm sugar or stevia, Smoothie Mix, and FiberMender. Blend until smooth and enjoy.

Strawberry Rhubarb Smoothie

Yields 1 serving

- ½ cup unsweetened coconut milk, like So Delicious, or use a different milk
- ¼ cup spinach
- 2 tablespoons frozen rhubarb (chop 1–2 stalks fresh rhubarb and freeze overnight if you can't find frozen rhubarb)
- ¼ cup frozen strawberries
- 1 teaspoon palm sugar or a pinch of stevia, plus more as needed
- 1 scoop All-in-One Vanilla Smoothie Mix (see Resources)
- 1 scoop FiberMender (see Resources)

Place coconut milk, spinach, rhubarb, and strawberries in blender. Blend until mostly combined. Add palm sugar or stevia, Smoothie Mix, and FiberMender. Blend until smooth and taste. Rhubarb can be very tart, so add another pinch of sugar or stevia, if needed.

6

CHAPTER SIX

BONE BROTH AND SOUP

There's something magical about making a batch of soup from scratch—cooking the bones into stock, preparing the mirepoix (see below), and stirring in the spices and add-ins until all of the simple ingredients come together to give you a nourishing, soothing brew.

MIREPOIX, SAY WHAT?

Pronounced *Meer-PWAH*, mirepoix is an essential ingredient in soups—one that you have probably used before without even knowing it has a fancy French name. Mirepoix is a combination of finely diced carrots, onion, and celery used to add aroma and flavor to stocks, soups, and sauces.

The ratio for a proper mirepoix is half onions and a quarter each celery and carrots. The smaller you chop your veggies, the quicker the stock will take on the flavor.

Cajuns call the combination a trinity and the Italians refer to it as soffritto. Whatever you call this combo of aromatics, a soup just isn't a soup without mirepoix.

Want a cool trick? For a colorless stock, swap out the carrots for parsnips.

As a general rule, use about a pound of mirepoix per five quarts of water.

BONE BROTH

Yes, I love soups. And since becoming a Part-Time Paleoista, I've made sure my soups start with bone broth. Bone broth is one of the most comforting, healing, and nutritious things you can make, and it's a staple in my house and in the homes of many Paleoistas—part-time or otherwise.

Bone broth is a stock made by simmering the bones of an animal (lamb, chicken, cow, pig) in water for several hours or even days. But it's much more than your basic soup stock.

Bone broths have been used medicinally in China for many, many years, and they are now being rightfully embraced, enthusiastically, by the Paleo crowd. Our grandmothers have always known that simmering leftover bones makes the best soups, haven't they?

Let's take a closer look at this magical elixir.

KEY BENEFITS OF BONE BROTH:

- **Strong teeth and bones.** All that good stuff from within the bones goes straight to your own bones and teeth, helping make them good and strong.
- **Greater gut health.** Leaky gut syndrome is becoming an epidemic in North America. Damage to the lining of the gut is caused by poor diet, chemicals, and toxins. Bone broth contains massive amounts of glutamine, which helps to heal your gut, plus the fats in the broth help us absorb the minerals.
- **Bone marrow.** When you consume bone broth made from good quality marrow bones, you're consuming bone marrow, which provides your body with many nutrients and healthy fats that balance and regulate hormones.
- **Joint health.** Bone broth has proteins in it—lots of them. One of those proteins is glucosamine, which a lot of people buy in pill form in the vitamin aisle to help ease joint pain.

HOW TO MAKE BONE BROTH

You'll be happy to know that bone broth is a snap to make. I make huge vats of the stuff all the time. Sometimes I make it with chicken carcasses after I've roasted a chicken or two (I save the carcasses in the freezer so I can do a big pot of them at a time). Or I'll use beef bones that I buy at the farmers' market. I get big bags of neck bones from grass-fed cows for next to nothing, roast them up, and make the most amazing bone broths.

Grass-fed animals are an important component of a good bone broth—remember, you eat what the animal you eat ate. In other words, whatever that cow ate, you get an opportunity to eat again, whether it's grass, chemicals, or hormones.

Take a big pot (or use your slow cooker) and put some roasted bones* into it. It's a good idea to mix your bones to get the most nutrition and flavor. Knuckle bones, neck bones, and foot bones are excellent in bone broths. I've made bone broth from chicken feet that is absolutely off-the-hook. Yes, that's right. Chicken feet. I have to tell you, staring at eight or so chicken feet floating in your slow cooker is a bit startling at first, but after making it just once, I always look for chicken feet at the farmers' market. The flavor is unbelievable and the nutrient value is better than that of a regular chicken carcass. I see you turning up your nose! But don't diss it till you try it.

So, you've got your bones in a pot. Now add whatever vegetables you want (I like onion, celery, carrots, garlic, and herbs). Cover with filtered water. Add a couple of tablespoons of apple cider vinegar to the pot. This is a critical ingredient to help coax the minerals and nutrients out of the bones.

Bring your broth to a boil on top of the stove or in a slow cooker and then let it simmer for at least twelve hours, but preferably for

---

* To roast bones, preheat oven to 350 degrees, drizzle bones with olive oil, sprinkle sea salt and freshly ground pepper over them, and roast for 15–20 minutes, or until nicely browned.

seventy-two hours. This is why I have two slow cookers! I can keep this going for a few days easily—it works great. Strain the broth when you've cooked it as long as you're going to.

You'll notice that once you've finished simmering your bones for hours and hours, you can actually push your fingernail into what was once a very hard bone. That is because all of those minerals that made the bones firm have been released into the liquid.

All of that calcium and phosphorous—the minerals that make up more than 60 percent of bone mass—will be going into your body when you eat the broth.

If you've done it just right, the broth should gelatinize when you refrigerate it overnight, just like a meat-flavored Jell-O. It's this gelatin that makes the broth so nutritious.

Reheat the broth and drink it plain if you want, use it in soups and sauces, turn it into a big pot of Mighty Mitochondria Soup . . . I don't care what you do with it, as long as you make it and consume it. If you want more exact measurements, here are some basic bone broth recipes to help get you started:

Beef Bone Broth

Yields approx. 7–8 cups

2 lbs roasted oxtails

2 lbs roasted beef knuckles or neck bones (whatever bones you can find)

7 cups water, plus more if needed

2 tablespoons apple cider vinegar

4 cloves garlic, pressed

2 yellow onions, halved

3 stalks celery, halved

2 leeks, trimmed and halved (or to fit in pot)

2 sprigs fresh rosemary

6 sprigs fresh oregano

6 sprigs fresh thyme

2 tablespoons whole peppercorns

1 teaspoon sea salt

In a large stockpot, place oxtails and other beef bones, add water, turn heat on high, and bring to a boil. Reduce heat to low, add apple cider vinegar, cover, and simmer for 1 hour. Add garlic, onions, celery, leeks, rosemary, oregano, thyme, peppercorns, and sea salt. Continue simmering uncovered for 5–6 hours, adding water 1 cup at a time, if needed. Strain the broth and cool completely, uncovered, discarding all bones, vegetables, and herbs.

This broth can also be made in a slow cooker (cooked on low for up to 72 hours).

Traditional Chicken Bone Broth

Yields approx. 7–8 cups

2 lbs roasted chicken backs

2 lbs roasted chicken feet

7 cups water, plus more if needed

3 cloves garlic, pressed

2 yellow onions, halved

3 stalks celery, halved

3 carrots, cut into 2-inch pieces

3 sprigs fresh rosemary

6 sprigs fresh oregano

6 sprigs fresh thyme

2 teaspoons whole peppercorns

1 teaspoon sea salt

2–3 tablespoons apple cider vinegar

In a large stockpot, place chicken backs and feet, add water, turn heat on high, and bring to a boil. Add garlic, onions, celery, carrots, rosemary, oregano, thyme, peppercorns, sea salt, and apple cider vinegar. Continue simmering uncovered for 3–4 hours, adding water 1 cup at a time, if needed. Strain the broth and cool completely, uncovered, discarding all bones, vegetables, and herbs.

Again, this whole batch can be done in a very large slow cooker and cooked for up to 2 days on low.

Simple Seafood Broth

Yields approx. 7–8 cups

5 cups shrimp shells, heads, and tails (from about 2 lbs shrimp)*
1 cup crab shells, crushed (from about ½ lb crab)*
1 cup lobster shells, crushed (3–4 lobster tails)*
2 tablespoons olive oil
3 cloves garlic, pressed
2 cups sliced leeks, white parts only
1 cup sliced celery
1 cup sliced scallions
7 cups water, plus more if needed
3 strips lemon peel, no pith
3 bay leaves
1 bunch Italian parsley
1 teaspoon sea salt
1 teaspoon whole peppercorns
2–3 tablespoons apple cider vinegar

Rinse heads and shells in cold water and drain. In a large stockpot, heat olive oil over medium heat. Add garlic, leeks, celery, and scallions, and sauté until leeks and celery become translucent and the other vegetables soften, about 7 minutes. Add heads and shells, and stir for a few seconds. Carefully add water, then lemon peel, bay leaves, parsley, sea salt, and peppercorns. Stir and bring to a boil, then reduce heat to low and simmer, uncovered, occasionally skimming the surface and discarding any foam.

Add apple cider vinegar before covering, and simmer for 45 minutes to an hour, adding water ¼ cup at a time, if needed, then removing from heat when a rich orange color develops. Strain, discarding shells, herbs, and vegetables. Cool completely, then refrigerate or freeze, if not using immediately.

You can also do this whole batch in the slow cooker for 8 hours on low, if you (a) have a big-enough slow cooker and (b) sauté everything first.

*Ask someone in the seafood department if they have the shrimp heads and the crab and lobster shells you need. You never know. If you have any trouble finding all these shells, just double up on what you do have—but you'll be very happy with the results if you have everything listed here.

SOUPS

Now that you're well schooled on the benefits of bone broth, what do you say we start making some actual soups? Here we go!

Mighty Mitochondria Soup

This soup is named as such because of Dr. Terry Wahls's influence on my nutritional life. The soup is chock-full of nutrients that will feed your mitochondria and make you healthy and strong.

Yields many servings!

3 tablespoons olive oil

3 large onions, chopped

3 large leeks, white parts only, chopped

6 cloves garlic (or more), pressed

3 large carrots, peeled and chopped

3 small stalks celery, chopped

1 medium turnip, peeled and chopped

2 huge leaves chard, de-ribbed and chopped

4 leaves each black kale and Scotch kale, de-ribbed and chopped

¼ head cabbage, chopped

2 small sweet potatoes, peeled and chopped

½ teaspoon dried thyme

Sea salt and freshly ground black pepper to taste

2 (14.5 oz) cans diced tomatoes, undrained

4 quarts bone broth

In a large soup pot, heat olive oil over medium-high heat; add onions and leeks and cook until nearly translucent. Add garlic and sauté for a couple of minutes, but don't let it brown. Add remaining fresh veggies and the sweet potatoes; sauté for just a minute or two. (You're not cooking them—just getting the wonderful flavor this quick step will infuse in your soup.) Add the thyme, sea salt, and pepper while sautéing.

Now place the veggies in a large slow cooker, and add diced tomatoes and broth. Cover and cook on low for 7–9 hours or on high for 4–6 hours (all slow cookers differ, depending on size, age, brand, etc.; your mileage may vary). If your slow cooker isn't large enough, simmer the mixture in the soup pot on the stove for at least 1 hour. Just before serving, gently mash some of the sweet potato chunks against the side of the slow cooker or soup pot to thicken the soup. Give it a stir and serve.

QUICK FIXES FOR SOUP VARIATIONS

Now, remember: Don't do these to the whole pot of soup—just the amount you pull out for each meal:

QUICK FIX #1: TEX-MEX VEGGIE SOUP

Add some salsa for a little heat (and a dash of cayenne, if you like), a little ground cumin, and chopped cilantro. Top with some diced avocado and more chopped cilantro.

QUICK FIX #2: TUSCAN VEGGIE SOUP

Add some fresh chopped basil leaves, chopped tomato, and cooked, gluten-free, and nitrate-free sausage.

QUICK FIX #3: AUTUMN VEGGIE SOUP

Add some cooked diced acorn or butternut squash, a sprinkling of ground nutmeg, and some chopped parsley. I also add an ample sprinkling of curry.

Mexican Wedding Soup

A new, ethnic spin on a traditional soup. You will love this!

Yields 6–8 servings

FIRST OFF, MAKE THE MEATBALLS:

¾ lb ground grass-fed beef

½ lb spicy Italian pork sausage, casings removed

⅓ cup almond meal

3 cloves garlic, pressed

4 tablespoons chopped cilantro

3 tablespoons almond milk

2 eggs, lightly beaten

Sea salt and freshly ground black pepper to taste

THEN THE SOUP PART:

2 tablespoons olive oil

1 large onion, finely chopped

3 carrots, chopped

2 stalks celery, chopped

10 cups bone broth (chicken or beef works)

½ cup dry white wine

¼ cup chopped cilantro

12 oz baby spinach

Garnishes: chopped cilantro and chopped avocado

Preheat the oven to 350 degrees. Place all meatball ingredients into a large mixing bowl. Using your clean hands, smoosh everything together well, and form the meatballs (about 1 ½ inches in diameter; you'll make about 34). Place them on a parchment-lined baking (jelly roll) pan and bake for 30 minutes. Set them aside when done.

While the meatballs are baking, start on the soup. In a large soup pot, heat olive oil over medium heat and add onion, carrots, and celery. Sauté till soft, about 5 minutes. Add bone broth and wine, and bring to a boil. Now add cilantro, meatballs, and spinach, heating for just a minute. Serve with more fresh cilantro over the top and some chopped avocado.

Seafood Chowder

Yields 6–8 servings

- 4 tablespoons coconut oil
- 2 medium onions, chopped
- 6 cloves garlic, pressed
- 4 medium stalks celery, chopped
- 2 medium carrots, peeled and chopped
- 2 ½ cups unsweetened coconut milk (canned or from a carton)
- 1 cup clam juice or seafood bone broth
- 4 cups chicken bone broth
- 2 medium turnips, peeled and chopped
- 2 teaspoons sea salt (or to taste)
- 1 ½ teaspoons ground white pepper
- 2 teaspoons dried thyme
- 3 lbs various seafood (shrimp, scallops, clams)
- 6 slices peppered bacon, cooked and chopped
- 2 tablespoons arrowroot starch
- 4 tablespoons water

Melt coconut oil in a large saucepan with a tight-fitting lid over medium-high heat. Add onions, garlic, celery, and carrots; cook and stir for 4 minutes or until onions are translucent. Stir in next 9 ingredients, then bring mixture to a low boil. Reduce heat to medium, cover, and cook for 8 minutes. Reduce heat to low and simmer for 10 minutes or until turnip is soft. In a small bowl or cup, combine arrowroot starch and water; stir into chowder, then bring to a slow boil and cook until slightly thickened. Serve.

Beefy Vegetable Soup

Yields 4–8 servings

    2 cups seeded, peeled, and diced butternut squash
    2 cups diced yellow onions
    1 cup sliced carrots
    2 cups chopped cauliflower
    2 cups chopped broccoli
    4 cups beef bone broth
    2 tablespoons lime juice
    5 cloves garlic, pressed
    1 tablespoon dried oregano
    ¼ teaspoon crushed red pepper flakes
    1 teaspoon sea salt
    ½ teaspoon freshly ground black pepper
    4 cups chopped Swiss chard

Place all ingredients except Swiss chard in a large slow cooker on low for 5–8 hours, until vegetables are fork tender. Stir in Swiss chard and continue to stir until nicely wilted. Serve!

Broccoli Soup

So easy—two ingredients and some salt and pepper, maybe a little thyme, if you like.

Yields 4–6 servings

    1 (16 oz) bag frozen broccoli
    4 cups bone broth (whatever kind you have on hand)

In a medium saucepan, empty the entire bag of frozen broccoli. Pour broth over the top. Heat till simmering and the broccoli is cooked through, about 5 minutes or so (depending on the size of the broccoli florets). Blend one batch at a time (fill up the blender only about halfway or it will make a huge mess). Then pour blended soup back into the pot; season with a little salt and pepper and some dried thyme, if you like. Ta-da! All done. It's a favorite lunchtime soup for me.

Curried Pumpkin and Shrimp Soup

Yields 6 servings

- 1 tablespoon olive oil
- 1 small onion, chopped
- 1 large garlic clove, pressed
- 3 cups chicken bone broth
- 1 cup canned coconut milk
- 3 cups pumpkin puree (not pumpkin pie filling)
- 2 teaspoons red curry paste
- Sea salt and pepper to taste
- 1 lb medium shrimp, peeled and deveined
- ¼ cup chopped cilantro

In a large pot, heat oil over medium-high heat. Add onion and garlic; sauté about 5 minutes, or until onion is translucent. Add bone broth, coconut milk, pumpkin puree, and red curry paste; simmer 15–20 minutes. Add sea salt and pepper to taste. Add shrimp and cover. Cook until shrimp is pink, about 5 minutes. Garnish with cilantro and serve.

Spicy Mexican Beef Soup

Yields 4 servings

- 2 tablespoons olive oil
- 1 cup chopped onion
- 6 cloves garlic, pressed
- ½ cup chopped cilantro

¼ cup lime juice

1 teaspoon lime zest

1 teaspoon chili powder

½ teaspoon ground cumin

4 ¾ cups beef bone broth

1 ½ lbs cooked cubed beef steak

1 cup chopped avocado

Heat oil in a large stockpot over medium heat. Add onion and garlic, and sauté until onion is translucent. Add cilantro, lime juice, and lime zest, stirring well. Add chili powder and cumin. Cook for 30 seconds, then add bone broth and beef-steak. Bring to a boil and cook for 15–20 minutes. Top each serving with ¼ cup avocado. Enjoy!

Sweet Onion and Mushroom Soup

Yields 4 servings

3 tablespoons olive oil

3 cups thickly sliced yellow onion

2 cups sliced baby bella mushrooms

3 cloves garlic, pressed

1 ½ tablespoons chopped fresh thyme

1 ½ tablespoons chopped fresh rosemary

¼ cup lemon juice

2 tablespoons tomato paste

5 cups beef bone broth, divided

Heat oil in a large stockpot over low heat. Add onion, mushrooms, garlic, and herbs. Cover and cook for 20 minutes. Stir well, and continue to cook for another hour and a half, checking every 30 minutes (when onions are a dark caramel color, you're ready to move on—it may take only an hour). Add lemon juice and tomato paste and stir well. Add about ½ cup broth; stir and scrape up any bits from the bottom. Stir in remaining broth, then cover and simmer for one more hour. When heated through, soup is ready to serve.

Creamy Sweet Potato Soup

Yields 4 servings

- 1 tablespoon coconut oil
- 4 cups chopped leeks
- 3 cups diced sweet potatoes
- ½ cup diced yellow onion
- 2 cloves garlic, pressed
- 5 cups chicken bone broth
- Sea salt and freshly ground black pepper to taste
- 4 (6 oz) boneless, skinless chicken thighs, cooked and cubed
- 2 cups unsweetened coconut milk (canned or from a carton)

In a large stockpot, heat coconut oil over medium-high heat. Cook leeks until soft and then bring sweet potato, onion, garlic, broth, sea salt, and pepper to a boil over medium-high heat. Stir well. As soon as broth comes to a boil, reduce heat to low and simmer until sweet potatoes are tender (10–15 minutes). Add chicken and coconut milk and heat through. Remove the soup from the heat and serve.

Chicken and Broccoli-Carrot Soup

Yields 4 servings

- 2 tablespoons olive oil
- 2 cups diced sweet onion
- 4 cloves garlic, pressed
- 1 tablespoon dried sage
- 1 cup canned coconut milk
- 4 cups chicken bone broth
- 4 cups chopped broccoli
- ½ cup diced carrots
- 1 teaspoon sea salt
- ½ teaspoon freshly ground black pepper

½ cup coconut cream

4 medium chicken breast halves, cooked and chopped

In a large stockpot, heat oil over medium heat. Add onion, garlic, and sage, and sauté until onion is translucent, 5–7 minutes. Carefully pour in coconut milk and broth, stirring to scrape up any bits from the bottom. Add broccoli, carrots, sea salt, and pepper, and bring to a boil. Reduce heat and simmer for 10–20 minutes, until vegetables are crisp-tender. Remove from heat.

Carefully pour half of the soup into a blender or food processor, and when cool, blend until smooth. Stir coconut cream and chicken into the pot, then return blended soup to pot and heat through over medium heat. Serve immediately after soup is heated through to avoid overcooking remaining vegetables, and enjoy!

Roasted Tomato Basil Bisque

Yields 4 servings

2 tablespoons olive oil

1 cup shallots or 1 small yellow onion, diced

4 cloves garlic, pressed

½ tablespoon dried thyme

1 teaspoon sea salt

½ teaspoon freshly ground black pepper

1 (14.5 oz) can diced roasted tomatoes, drained

2 cups tomato sauce

1 cup chicken bone broth

¼ cup chopped fresh basil

In a large stockpot, heat oil over medium heat. Add shallots, garlic, and spices, and sauté until shallots are translucent, 5–7 minutes. Carefully pour in diced tomatoes, tomato sauce, and broth, stirring to scrape up any bits from the bottom.

Bring to a boil, then reduce heat and simmer for 10–20 minutes, until heated through. Remove from heat. Serve as is, if you like a chunky texture, or blend in batches in a blender or food processor when cooled, then return blended soup to pot and heat through over medium heat. Stir in chopped basil, serve immediately, and enjoy!

Part-Time Paleo Tip: Sprinkle the top with Parmigiano-Reggiano.

Coconut Shrimp Soup with Zucchini "Noodles"

Yields 4–6 servings

2 cups chicken bone broth
3 tablespoons fish sauce
3 tablespoons lime juice
1 tablespoon grated ginger
2 cloves garlic, pressed
1 tablespoon raw honey
½ teaspoon crushed red pepper flakes
¼ teaspoon ground coriander
1 cup chopped bell pepper
12 oz zucchini "noodles" (use a vegetable peeler to make long strips)
1 ½ cups canned coconut milk
1 lb medium shrimp, peeled and deveined
½ cup chopped cilantro
2 tablespoons sliced green onions

In a large stockpot, heat broth, fish sauce, lime juice, ginger, garlic, honey, red pepper flakes, ground coriander, and bell pepper over medium heat. Bring to a boil, then immediately stir in zucchini noodles and coconut milk. Reduce heat and simmer for 5–7 minutes. Stir in shrimp and cook for another 2–3 minutes, until pink and cooked through. Stir in cilantro and green onions. Serve immediately.

Crab and Avocado Gazpacho

Yields 4–6 servings

2 avocados, chopped

1 (14.5 oz) can diced tomatoes

1 cup chopped red onion

2 cloves garlic, pressed

2 tablespoons lime juice

¼ cup chopped cilantro

1 cup coconut milk from a carton, chilled

¾ cup clam juice, chilled

½ cup cold water

1 tablespoon lemon juice

1 lb lump crabmeat

1 teaspoon sea salt

½ teaspoon freshly ground black pepper or to taste

In a food processor, combine avocados, tomatoes, onion, garlic, lime juice, and cilantro. Pulse until mostly smooth but still a bit chunky. Set aside. In a large bowl, combine coconut milk, clam juice, water, lemon juice, and crabmeat. Stir well. Scrape the avocado mixture into the crab mixture and stir until well combined. Season with salt and pepper, cover tightly, and chill in the fridge for 30 minutes. Serve cold and enjoy.

Hearty Chicken Vegetable Noodle Soup

Yields 4–6 servings

2 tablespoons olive oil

½ cup chopped yellow onion

2 cloves garlic, pressed

1 teaspoon dried sage

1 cup sliced carrots

1 cup frozen green beans, cut in half (don't use French style)

4 cups chicken bone broth

2 cups chopped kale

1 lb boneless, skinless chicken thigh meat, cubed

1 teaspoon sea salt

½ teaspoon freshly ground black pepper or to taste

1 (16 oz) package fresh kelp noodles, rinsed (you can find them in a health food store)

In a large stockpot, heat oil over medium heat. Add onion, garlic, sage, and carrots. Cook for 7–10 minutes, until onion is translucent and carrots are becoming tender.

Carefully add green beans and broth, stirring and scraping up any bits that may be on the bottom. Add kale, chicken, sea salt, and pepper. Bring to a boil, then reduce heat and simmer for 4–7 minutes, until the kale wilts and chicken is cooked. Add kelp noodles and cook an additional minute. Serve immediately.

Coconut Beef Curry Soup

Yields 4–6 servings

2 tablespoons coconut oil

2 lbs beef stew meat

Sea salt and pepper to taste

1 cup thickly sliced carrots

4 cups coconut milk from a carton

1 tablespoon red curry paste

2 cups beef bone broth

2 cups cubed sweet potatoes

2 cups chopped baby bok choy

1 (8 oz) package fresh kelp noodles, rinsed

In a large stockpot, heat oil over medium-high heat. Brown meat on all sides, adding sea salt and pepper to taste. Add carrots, and continue to cook until they start to caramelize. Add coconut milk, red curry paste, broth, sweet potatoes, and bok choy. Bring to a simmer and cook for 30–45 minutes, or until sweet potatoes are tender. Add kelp noodles and continue to cook until heated through. Serve right away.

Italian Chicken Meatball Soup

Yields 4–6 servings

1 lb ground chicken
1 teaspoon dried basil
1 teaspoon dried oregano
1 clove garlic, pressed
2 tablespoons olive oil
2 cups tomato sauce
3 cups chicken bone broth
1 cup chopped onion
1 cup chopped red bell pepper
1 cup chopped leeks
3 cloves garlic, pressed
1 teaspoon sea salt
½ teaspoon freshly ground black pepper
1 tablespoon dried basil
1 cup chopped button mushrooms

In a medium bowl, combine ground chicken, basil, oregano, and garlic. Make 1-inch meatballs until all of the meat is used. In a large stockpot, heat oil over medium-high heat. Brown meatballs on all sides. In a large bowl, combine tomato sauce, broth, onion, red bell pepper, leeks, garlic, sea salt, pepper, and basil. Pour over meatballs. Cover and cook on low for 45–60 minutes. Turn heat to medium-high and add mushrooms, stirring well, then re-cover and cook for another 15–20 minutes, until mushrooms are cooked through. Serve immediately and enjoy!

Soup is a terrific option for eating Paleo. But what else are you going to eat? Time to take a good, close look at some different Paleo meal plans. In the next chapter, you'll get four weeks' worth of meals, with three meals a day, all laid out for you. I really couldn't make this any easier, people—now, let's get going.

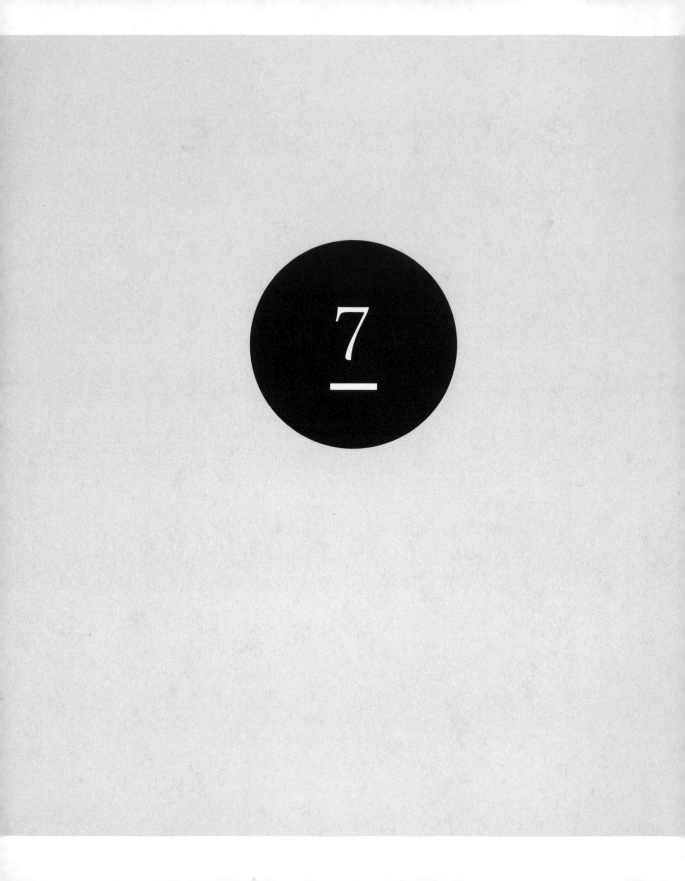

7

CHAPTER SEVEN
PALEO MENU PLANS

P lanning your meals can be a daunting task, even for the überorganized. At first, it's fun. Then it gets frustrating and, about an hour into it, you want to toss your cookbooks, computer, and everything else you have onto the front lawn and call for a pizza.

Throw this new Paleo stuff into the mix and you find yourself in pretty deep. It's scary—you don't know how to proceed and you think you're doomed to a life of kale and steak for breakfast, lunch, and dinner.

This is why a lot of people give up after about a week and go back to what they know. The task of menu planning can be simply too overwhelming for a lot of folks.

Whether you want to do menu planning yourself or not, I want to teach you a few good skills for putting your meal plans together. I know meal planning. *Reader's Digest* called me "the Mother of Meal Planning." You could say I've made my name in the meal-planning space. In fact, SavingDinner.com is the original meal-planning website (before we were SavingDinner.com, we were MenuMailer.net, started in 2001). Before then, there were really no meal-planning websites.

You have to start with the basics of what your meals will look like. Breakfast can be as uncomplicated as a smoothie. That is my top recommendation—it is simple (plus it's an easy to-go option for your commute or carpool) and has all the nutrients needed to start strong right out of the gate. But if you'd prefer to have a bowl of beef stew for breakfast, go right ahead.

Personally, I like to keep lunch simple, too. Having a vat of Mighty Mitochondria Soup on hand in the fridge makes for a quick lunch. I simply add some chopped protein from the night before, and presto—instant lunch after the soup is warmed up a bit. Add a salad, and now you'll be hitting it out of the park, nutrient-wise.

I throw a slow cooker meal in every week. There's always one day out of the week when throwing something in that marvelous appliance will save your sanity. There's nothing quite like a slow cooker. It's like coming home to a personal chef. You smell dinner as you walk in the door, and ah—just like that, your stress melts away!

I've handed you a full month's worth of meals here that you can use over and over again as you get used to this new, Part-Time Paleo lifestyle. These plans include a weekly shopping list (written for a family of four) and daily recipes. Breakfast, lunch, and dinner are all planned out for you.

There are a few recipes you're going to find yourself leaning on time and time again when you adopt your Part-Time Paleo lifestyle. You will be tempted to boil up potatoes or pasta if you don't have some good basic side dishes in your arsenal.

STANDARD PART-TIME PALEO SIDE DISHES

These dishes come naturally to me now that I've made them each a gazillion times, and they will eventually come naturally to you, too.

Blue Spinach Salad

6 handfuls baby spinach

1 cup chopped walnuts

2 tablespoons balsamic vinegar

6 tablespoons extra virgin olive oil

1 ½ cups fresh blueberries

½ cup thinly sliced red onion

In a salad bowl, place the spinach down first, and then add the rest of the ingredients. Toss well and serve.

Leanne's Basic Vinaigrette

½ tablespoon Dijon mustard

1 ½ tablespoons balsamic vinegar

½ tablespoon lemon juice

1 small clove garlic, pressed

⅓ cup olive oil

Pepper to taste

Whisk all ingredients together. This vinaigrette goes well with any greens you have in the fridge.

Mashed Faux-Tatoes

1 medium head cauliflower, chopped

2 tablespoons butter

2 tablespoons cream cheese

salt and pepper to taste

Chop cauliflower into bite-size pieces and steam until you can easily pierce them with a fork. Drain the water off, and pat the cauliflower with a clean towel

to remove excess moisture. Put the cauliflower in your blender or food processor and blend with butter, cream cheese, salt, and pepper for a delicious side
dish.

Cauliflower "Rice"

1 medium head cauliflower, chopped
Salt and pepper to taste

Process raw cauliflower in a food processor or blender until it resembles grains
of rice. Steam "rice" until tender; drain. Add salt and pepper to taste, and fluff
with a fork. From here, you can get as creative as you like (see the Fried "Rice"
Recipe on page 111 for an example).

WEEK ONE SHOPPING LIST

Items marked with an asterisk (*) denote those needed for suggested
side dishes and are, therefore, optional for the week's menu plan. Quantities will vary, depending on how often you choose to serve the suggested dish.

PROTEIN

- Eggs (48; 2 hard-boiled in advance)
- Bacon (20 strips)
- Peeled and deveined shrimp (1 lb)
- Sliced cold-cut turkey (2 lbs)
- Smoked cold-cut ham (½ lb)
- Boneless, skinless chicken breast halves (14 medium)
- New York strip steaks (or cut of your choice), 6 oz (4)
- Sausage (5 oz)

- Kielbasa sausage (1 large link)
- Halibut fillets, 6 oz (7)
- Salmon fillets, 6 oz (4)
- Boneless pork chops, 6 oz (4)
- Prosciutto (8 slices)

CONDIMENTS

- Ghee
- Coconut oil
- Olive oil
- Raw honey
- Coconut aminos (see Resources)
- Rice vinegar
- Apple cider vinegar
- Red wine vinegar
- Dijon mustard
- Vanilla extract
- Olives*

SPICES

- Sea salt
- Black peppercorns
- Red pepper flakes
- Rosemary
- Paprika
- Garlic powder
- Onion powder
- Cinnamon
- Cayenne pepper
- Chili powder

PRODUCE

- Sweet potatoes (5)
- Red onions (3 ½)
- Garlic (27 cloves)
- Cucumbers (3)
- Avocados (3)
- Okra (1 ½ cups chopped)
- Roma tomatoes (3)
- Large tomatoes (3)
- Yellow onions (5)
- Jalapeño (1)
- Mango (1)
- Pineapple (1)
- Radishes (6)
- Celery (2 stalks)
- Cherry tomatoes (handful)
- Red bell peppers (4)
- Yellow bell peppers (2)
- Green bell pepper (1)
- Butter lettuce leaves, or other large-leaf lettuce (24)
- Romaine lettuce (2 cups)
- Mixed baby greens (6 cups)
- Spinach (5 cups)
- Carrots (2)
- Lime (1)
- Lemon (1)
- Cauliflower (1 head)
- Fresh thyme (1 tablespoon)
- Fresh parsley (2 tablespoons)
- Salad greens* (your choice of dark greens—no iceberg lettuce!)
- Salad goodies* (whatever you like: slivered almonds, raisins, chopped onions, etc.)

- Broccoli*
- Cauliflower*
- Green beans*
- Asparagus*
- Carrots*

CANNED GOODS

- Unsweetened coconut milk (in a carton, 2 tablespoons)
- Low-sodium chicken broth (4 cups)
- Unsweetened pureed pumpkin—not pumpkin pie filling (14 oz)

DRY GOODS

- Raw cashews (1 ¾ cups)
- Raw almonds (½ cup)
- Unsweetened shredded coconut (½ cup)
- Dried figs (4)
- Unsweetened dried cranberries (¼ cup)

FREEZER

- Orange juice concentrate (4 tablespoons)

OTHER

- Toothpicks
- Wooden skewers
- White wine

WEEK ONE RECIPES

DAY ONE

Breakfast: Sweet Potato Scramble

Yields 4 servings

   8 large eggs, whisked
   1 tablespoon coconut oil
   1 sweet potato, peeled and diced
   ½ red onion, chopped
   2 cloves garlic, pressed
   Sea salt and freshly ground black pepper to taste

Heat coconut oil in a large skillet over medium-high heat. Once oil is melted, add sweet potato, red onion, and garlic. Stir regularly for about 8 minutes (or until sweet potato starts to soften). Turn heat down to medium, pour whisked eggs into the pan, and stir until cooked through (about 3–5 minutes). Season with salt and pepper and serve!

Lunch: Paleo California Club Sandwich

Yields 4 servings

   8 large butter lettuce leaves
   Dijon mustard
   1 cucumber, sliced
   1 avocado, sliced
   1 large tomato, sliced
   ½ yellow onion, sliced
   4 strips bacon (my favorite is peppered), cut in half and cooked

½ lb–1 lb your favorite cold-cut turkey (make sure to read ingredients to
   avoid processed cold cuts)
Sea salt and freshly ground pepper

Sandwiches are pretty self-explanatory, and you can either make the family a
bunch or put out all the ingredients and let everyone fend for themselves. Consider your lettuce leaves your bread: Spread a little mustard on one or both sides
and then start layering the cucumber, avocado, tomato, onion, bacon, and turkey. Top it off with a dash of salt and pepper and your lunch is served (also a
great lunch for on-the-go).

Dinner: Honeyed Cashew Chicken

Yields 4 servings

   ¼ cup raw honey
   1 ½ tablespoons coconut aminos
   2 cloves garlic, pressed
   1 teaspoon sea salt
   1 teaspoon crushed red pepper flakes
   6 boneless, skinless chicken breast halves
   1 cup finely chopped raw cashews
   1–2 tablespoons ghee

   Note: This recipe uses 4 chicken breast halves—the extra 2 are to be used for Day
   Two's lunch.

In a medium bowl, whisk together first five ingredients. Dip each chicken breast
half into the mixture, making sure all sides are evenly coated. After soaking one,
sprinkle with cashews on all sides. Repeat with remaining chicken. Heat ghee in
a large skillet over medium-high heat and sear chicken for 4–6 minutes per side,
or until cooked through.
   Serving suggestion: Steamed kale and/or a large green salad

DAY TWO

Breakfast: Bacon Fried Eggs

Yields 4 servings

    8 strips of your favorite bacon
    8 large eggs
    Sea salt and freshly ground black pepper to taste

This recipe is so easy and delicious. First, in a large skillet over medium-high heat, cook your bacon (roughly 3–6 minutes per side, or however you like your bacon cooked). Once bacon is done cooking, remove from pan, pour grease into a small bowl, then heat another skillet over medium-high heat. Add a table-spoon or two of bacon grease to the pan and crack a couple of eggs in (I usually like to do two at a time). For a great over-medium yolk consistency, let the eggs cook for 1–2 minutes, until you see the bottom side of the white start to cook through, and then, with a spatula, flip the eggs and fry on the other side for 1–2 minutes. Season eggs with salt and pepper and serve with bacon.

Lunch: Asian Accented Salad

Yields 4 servings

    SALAD:

    2 cups romaine lettuce
    2 cups spinach
    ¼ cup shredded carrots
    1 cucumber, sliced
    ½ red onion, chopped
    ¼ cup chopped raw cashews
    2 boneless, skinless chicken breast halves, cooked and chopped
        (leftover from Day One's dinner)

VINAIGRETTE:

¾ cup olive oil

3 cloves garlic, pressed

1 teaspoon sea salt

1 teaspoon freshly ground black pepper

2 tablespoons coconut aminos

1 tablespoon raw honey

¼ cup rice vinegar

In a large serving bowl, toss together all ingredients for the salad. Then in a medium bowl, thoroughly whisk together vinaigrette ingredients. Add one or two tablespoons of vinaigrette to a serving of salad, and lunch is served.

Dinner: Mustard-Rubbed Steak

Yields 4 servings

2 tablespoons olive oil

2 tablespoons Dijon mustard

1 tablespoon raw honey

3 tablespoons apple cider vinegar

4 cloves garlic, pressed

1 teaspoon sea salt

1 teaspoon freshly ground black pepper

4 (6 oz) New York Strip steaks (or cut of your choice)

In a medium bowl, whisk together all ingredients except steaks. Place steaks in a large zipper-style plastic bag and pour mixture inside. Seal and refrigerate for 4 hours or overnight. Before cooking, preheat grill to medium-high. Remove steaks from marinade and grill for 4–6 minutes per side or until cooked according to your preference (depending on thickness of steaks).

Serving suggestion: Roasted sweet potatoes and sautéed green beans

DAY THREE

Breakfast: Spinach and Sausage "Quiche"

Yields 4 servings

  1 cup spinach
  5 oz (1 cup), cooked sausage (if you can, try local sausage—
    your farmers' market or health food store should have some)
  8 large eggs, cracked into a bowl and whisked
  1 teaspoon sea salt
  1 teaspoon freshly ground black pepper
  1 teaspoon paprika
  ½ teaspoon dried rosemary
  1 tablespoon ghee, melted

Preheat oven to 350 degrees.

In a large bowl, mix all ingredients except ghee. Pour ghee into a pie pan or baking dish, and use a paper towel to spread on all sides of dish. Pour egg mixture into dish and bake for 30–40 minutes or until cooked through.

Lunch: Radish Stacks

Yields 4 servings

  4–6 radishes, sliced
  1 cucumber, sliced
  1 avocado, diced
  1 large handful cherry tomatoes
  ½ lb–1 lb cold-cut turkey
  Dijon mustard (optional)
  Toothpicks or skewers

This is a fun little lunch, especially if you have kids—they'll get a kick out of it. Assemble all the ingredients, kebab-style, on a toothpick or skewer, alternating veggies and turkey (I usually fold the turkey, then stick it on, or cut it into smaller pieces). I like to dip the stacks in a little mustard, but they're also good plain.

Dinner: White Wine–Glazed Halibut

Yields 4 servings

⅓ cup white wine

3 tablespoons raw honey

1 tablespoon Dijon mustard

1 teaspoon sea salt

1 teaspoon freshly ground black pepper

½ teaspoon garlic powder

½ teaspoon onion powder

6–7 (6 oz) halibut fillets (or other firm white fish)

2 tablespoons ghee

Note: This recipe uses 4 halibut fillets—the extra 2–3 are to be used for Day Four's lunch.

In a medium bowl, whisk together all ingredients except fish and ghee. Brush mixture over all sides of each fillet. Heat ghee in a large skillet over medium-high heat and sear fish for 3–4 minutes per side or until cooked through.

Serving suggestion: Steamed carrots, broccoli, and cauliflower

DAY FOUR

Breakfast: Honey Butter Sweet Potato Hash

Yields 4 servings

- 8 slices bacon
- 1 sweet potato, peeled and shredded (use cheese grater)
- 3 tablespoons ghee, melted and divided
- 2 tablespoons raw honey
- 8 eggs, cracked into a bowl and whisked
- Sea salt and freshly ground black pepper to taste

Preheat oven to 375 degrees.

Cook bacon. In a large bowl, place grated sweet potato. In a small bowl, whisk together 2 tablespoons of melted ghee and honey. Pour over sweet potato and toss to coat. Spread out on a cookie sheet and bake for 10–15 minutes (watch it closely to make sure it doesn't burn). Heat the remaining tablespoon of ghee in a large skillet over medium-high heat. Pour eggs in skillet, season with salt and pepper, and scramble. Stir and cook for about 5 minutes or until cooked through. Serve with hash and bacon.

Lunch: Fish Tacos with Mango Salsa

Yields 4 servings

TACOS:

- 2–3 (6 oz) halibut or other white fish fillets, cooked and chopped (leftover from Day Three's dinner)
- 8 large lettuce leaves, such as butter lettuce
- 1 tablespoon coconut oil
- 1 yellow onion, chopped

1 red bell pepper, sliced

1 yellow bell pepper, sliced

MANGO SALSA:

1 large mango, peeled and chopped

2 tablespoons raw honey

1 jalapeño, seeded and chopped

½ red onion, chopped

3 roma tomatoes, chopped

1 teaspoon sea salt

1 tablespoon lime juice

Place a handful of fish in each lettuce leaf (aka your taco shells). Heat coconut oil in a large skillet over medium-high heat and sauté onion and bell peppers. Cook for 5–8 minutes, stirring regularly until onion is translucent and peppers are soft. Place a handful of onion and peppers on top of fish in lettuce. Place all salsa ingredients in a food processor. Pulse until all ingredients are well blended. Serve salsa on top of tacos.

Dinner: Tangy Soaked Pork

Yields 4 servings

⅓ cup apple cider vinegar

2 tablespoons olive oil

1 tablespoon raw honey

2 tablespoons coconut aminos

4 cloves garlic, pressed

1 teaspoon sea salt

1 teaspoon crushed red pepper flakes

4 (6 oz) boneless pork chops

In a medium bowl, whisk together all ingredients except pork. Place pork in a large zipper-style bag, pour mixture inside, seal bag, and marinate in refrigerator for 4 hours or overnight. Before cooking, preheat grill to medium-high. Remove pork from marinade and grill for 4–6 minutes per side or until cooked through.

Serving suggestion: A large green salad is all you'll need!

DAY FIVE

Breakfast: Eggs Florentine

Yields 4 servings

1 tablespoon apple cider vinegar
4–8 slices prosciutto (depending on how much your family eats)
1 tablespoon ghee
2 cloves garlic, pressed
½ yellow onion, chopped
2 cups spinach
1 large tomato, sliced
8 eggs
Sea salt and freshly ground black pepper to taste

Preheat oven to 375 degrees. Fill a pot halfway with water, add apple cider vinegar, and bring almost to a boil. While water heats, place prosciutto on a cookie sheet and bake in oven for 5–10 minutes (or until crispy). Heat ghee in a large skillet over medium-high heat. Add garlic, onion, and spinach. Sauté for 2–5 minutes, until spinach wilts. Remove from heat.

Divide spinach mixture among 4 plates. Place prosciutto and tomato on top.

Once water just begins to boil, reduce heat to a strong simmer. Crack one egg into a small bowl, make sure yolk is intact, and slowly slide it into the simmering water. Wait for 2–4 minutes, until white is set (they will be opaque; they're about done if you like them medium-runny). Use a slotted spoon to remove egg from water. Continue with the rest of the eggs.

On each prepared plate, serve two eggs on top of spinach mixture. Season to taste with salt and pepper.

Lunch: Cobb Salad Wraps

Yields 4 servings

Dijon mustard

8 large lettuce leaves

2 hard-boiled eggs, peeled and chopped

2 chicken breast halves, cooked and chopped

1 large tomato, chopped

1 avocado, chopped

½ lb smoked cold-cut ham

Leanne's Basic Vinaigrette (recipe on page 95)

To prepare wraps, spread mustard on inside of lettuce leaves, layer remaining ingredients, and drizzle with vinaigrette; then, roll up like a wrap—makes a great on-the-go lunch.

Dinner: Sweet and Sour Chicken Pineapple Kebabs

Yields 4 servings

SAUCE:

2 tablespoons raw honey

4 tablespoons coconut aminos

2 teaspoons red wine vinegar

1 tablespoon olive oil

1 teaspoon sea salt

1 teaspoon cinnamon

KEBABS:

4 boneless, skinless chicken breast halves, cubed

1 red bell pepper, cut into large chunks

1 yellow bell pepper, cut into large chunks

1 red onion, chopped into large chunks

1 pineapple, cut into chunks

Wooden skewers (soak in water for 30 minutes so they won't catch fire)

Note: This recipe uses 3 chicken breast halves. The extra breast can be used in Day Six's lunch.

Preheat outdoor grill to medium-high. Whisk together sauce ingredients in a medium bowl. Then, on skewers, alternate ingredients for kebabs. Saturate kebabs with sauce and grill for 4–6 minutes per side or until cooked through.

Serving suggestion: Stir-fried vegetables (whatever you have in your crisper) and some Cauliflower "Rice" if you like

DAY SIX

Breakfast: Paleo Granola

Yields 4 servings

½ cup raw almonds

½ cup raw cashews

½ cup unsweetened shredded coconut

4 dried figs, chopped

¼ cup unsweetened dried cranberries

2 tablespoons orange juice concentrate

⅓ cup raw honey

3 tablespoons ghee, melted

1 teaspoon vanilla extract

½ teaspoon sea salt

Preheat oven to 300 degrees. In a food processor, lightly pulse almonds and cashews, just to get them slightly chopped. Place them in a large bowl and add coconut, figs, and cranberries. In a small bowl, whisk together orange juice, honey, ghee, vanilla, and salt. Pour over dry mixture, and mix well until fully coated. Spread out on a large cookie sheet and bake for 20–25 minutes or until everything is lightly browned and crunchy. Eat plain or in a bowl with some coconut or almond milk.

Lunch: Fried "Rice"

Yields 4 servings

- 2 tablespoons coconut oil
- 1 yellow onion, chopped
- 1 green bell pepper, sliced
- 1 red bell pepper, sliced
- 3 cloves garlic, pressed
- 1 head cauliflower, steamed to crisp texture (be sure it's not overcooked and mushy)
- 2 eggs
- 2 tablespoons coconut aminos
- 1 teaspoon sea salt
- 1 teaspoon crushed red pepper flakes
- 1 cup meat of your choice, cooked and cubed (leftovers from Day Five's dinner would work well, or any leftover meat you have)

Heat coconut oil in large wok over medium-high heat. Add onion, bell peppers, and garlic. Sauté for about 2 minutes to let onion sweat and become transparent, stirring occasionally. Meanwhile, place cauliflower in a food processor and pulse until nearly minced and almost the consistency of rice. Add cauliflower rice to wok. Move rice and veggies to one side of the wok, and crack the eggs into the other side. Take a spatula and start stirring quickly, scrambling the eggs and mixing with the rest of the food, while getting the cauliflower rice nice and fried on all sides. Right before you remove from heat, add remaining ingredients, including meat. Stir a few more times and then serve.

Dinner: Island Seasoned Salmon

Yields 4 servings

 1 teaspoon sea salt

 1 teaspoon freshly ground black pepper

 1 teaspoon paprika

 ½ teaspoon cayenne pepper

 ½ teaspoon chili powder

 ½ teaspoon garlic powder

 ¼ teaspoon onion powder

 ¼ teaspoon crushed red pepper flakes

 ¼ teaspoon cinnamon

 2 tablespoons raw honey

 1 tablespoon orange juice concentrate

 1 teaspoon apple cider vinegar

 4 (6 oz) salmon fillets

 1 tablespoon coconut oil

In a small bowl, combine all spices. In a separate small bowl, whisk together honey, orange juice, and vinegar. Brush the honey mixture on all sides of each fillet. Then, season all fillets evenly with spice mix. Heat coconut oil in a large skillet over medium-high heat and sear each fillet for 2–4 minutes per side or until cooked through.

 Serving suggestion: Steamed broccoli and Cauliflower "Rice"

DAY SEVEN

Breakfast: Sweet Potato Hash with Poached Eggs

Yields 4 servings

 3 large sweet potatoes, cubed and steamed

 1 yellow onion, chopped

2 tablespoons ghee, melted

3 cloves garlic, minced

1 tablespoon chopped fresh thyme

1 teaspoon sea salt

½ teaspoon freshly ground black pepper

4 eggs

2 tablespoons chopped parsley

Preheat oven to 400 degrees. In a large bowl, toss together everything but eggs and parsley. Place mixture on a parchment-lined sheet pan and cook for 15–20 minutes (tossing several times) or until sweet potatoes are golden brown. Meanwhile, poach the eggs. Evenly arrange hash on plates. Sprinkle with a little chopped parsley, then top with a poached egg and serve.

Lunch: Wilted Greens with Lemon Shrimp

Yields 4 servings

2 tablespoons coconut oil

1 large red bell pepper, chopped

1 red onion, chopped

1 clove garlic, pressed

1 lb shrimp, peeled and deveined

6 cups mixed baby greens

2 tablespoons unsweetened coconut milk

1 lemon, juice and zest

1 teaspoon sea salt

½ teaspoon freshly ground black pepper

Melt coconut oil in a large skillet over medium-high heat. Add bell pepper, onion, and garlic; cook until onion is soft. Add shrimp and cook, turning once, for 2–4 minutes, or until pink and opaque. Add greens; cook until wilted. Add coconut milk, then season with lemon juice and zest, salt, and pepper. Remove from heat and serve.

Dinner: Chicken Pumpkin Stew

Serves 4

4 cups low-sodium chicken broth, or use homemade

1 (14 oz) can unsweetened pureed pumpkin (not pumpkin pie filling)

2 boneless, skinless chicken breast halves, cubed

1 large link kielbasa sausage, chopped

1 yellow onion, chopped

3 cloves garlic, pressed

2 medium stalks celery, chopped

1 carrot, chopped

1 ½ cups chopped okra

1 teaspoon sea salt

1 teaspoon freshly ground black pepper

1 teaspoon cayenne pepper

½ teaspoon paprika

½ teaspoon ground cinnamon

In a large bowl, whisk together broth and pumpkin. Pour mixture into a large slow cooker, and then add remaining ingredients. Stir to blend well. Cover and cook on low for 8–10 hours, stirring every few hours.

Serving suggestion: Serve over Cauliflower "Rice"; add braised collard greens on the side.

WEEK TWO SHOPPING LIST

Items marked with an asterisk (*) denote those needed for suggested side dishes and are, therefore, optional for the week's menu plan. Quantities will vary, depending on how often you choose to serve the suggested dish.

PROTEIN

- Sliced cold-cut turkey breast (1 lb + 8 slices)
- Whole chicken (4–6 lbs)
- Boneless, skinless chicken breast halves (5 medium)
- Bacon (17 slices, 4–6 of those should be thick sliced)
- Canadian bacon (17 slices)
- Eggs (43; hard-boil 16 in advance)
- Ground turkey (1 ½ lbs)
- London broil (2 lbs)
- Boneless pork chops (4)
- Peeled and deveined shrimp (2 lbs + 2 cups)
- Crabmeat (18 oz)
- Filet mignon (1 lb)

CONDIMENTS

- Apple cider vinegar
- Ghee
- Coconut oil
- Avocado oil
- Olive oil
- White wine vinegar
- Balsamic vinegar
- Dijon mustard
- Raw honey
- Almond butter
- Vanilla extract
- Pure maple syrup

SPICES

- Sea salt
- Black peppercorns
- Cumin
- Red pepper flakes
- Cayenne pepper
- Chili powder
- Cinnamon
- Dried thyme
- Dried rosemary
- Onion powder
- Garlic powder
- Paprika

PRODUCE

- Spinach (1 cup)
- Sweet potatoes (3, plus serving suggestion)
- Cauliflower (5 cups chopped)
- Baby spinach (6 cups)
- Banana (2–3)
- Sprouts (1 cup)
- Cucumbers (2)
- Strawberries (1 cup)
- Radishes (10)
- Lemons (4)
- Limes (2)
- Yellow onions (4)
- Red onions (3)
- Parsley (½ cup chopped)
- Garlic (28 cloves)
- Vine-ripened tomatoes (10)

- Green bell peppers (3)
- Green onions (¼ cup chopped)
- Red cabbage (½ cup chopped)
- Orange (1)
- Celery (5 stalks)
- Blueberries (½ cup)
- Avocados (6)
- Lettuce leaves (24)
- Kale (1 cup)
- Carrots (2)
- Poblano peppers (3)
- Jalapeños (2)
- Fresh cilantro (4 handfuls)
- Salad greens* (your choice of dark greens—no iceberg lettuce!)
- Salad goodies* (whatever you like: slivered almonds, raisins, chopped onions, etc.)
- Cauliflower*
- Broccoli*
- Peppers*
- Butternut squash*
- Parsnips*
- Cabbage*
- Green beans*
- Bok choy*
- Carrots*
- Asparagus*

CANNED GOODS

- Unsweetened coconut milk (in a carton, 2 ¾ cups)
- Unsweetened almond milk (2 cups)
- Salsa verde (2 14-oz jars + 1 cup)
- Low-sodium chicken broth (6 cups)

DRY GOODS

- Cacao nibs (4 tablespoons)
- All-in-One Smoothie Mix, any flavor (2 scoops, see Resources)
- All-in-One Chai Smoothie Mix (8 scoops)
- Unsweetened cranberries (¼ cup)
- Almond meal (¾ cup)
- Almonds (1 cup slivered; ¼ cups chopped)
- Arrowroot starch

DAIRY

- Butter*

FREEZER

- Raspberries (½ cup)
- Bananas (2)
- Cherries (1 ½ cups)

OTHER

- Wooden skewers
- Red wine
- White wine

WEEK TWO RECIPES

DAY ONE

Breakfast: Paleo Power Smoothie

Yields 4 servings

- 12 ice cubes
- 2 scoops All-in-One Smoothie Mix
- 1–2 cups coconut milk (more can be used if smoothie is too thick)
- 1 cup spinach
- ½ cup frozen raspberries
- ½ cup frozen cherries
- 2 tablespoons cacao nibs

Place all ingredients in a blender and blend until smooth. (The thickness will depend on the amount of coconut milk, so feel free to add more or less, according to how you like your smoothie.)

Lunch: California Kebabs

Serves 4

- 4–6 thick slices of bacon
- 2–3 vine-ripened tomatoes, quartered
- 2 avocados, cut into large chunks
- 1 lb sliced cold-cut turkey breast
- 6 radishes, quartered
- Wooden skewers
- 1 lemon, quartered
- Sea salt and freshly ground black pepper to taste

Cook bacon soft, not crisp.

Alternate tomatoes, avocados, turkey, bacon, and radishes on the skewers. Lightly spritz with lemon, and season with salt and pepper. Serve.

Dinner: Tomatillo Shredded Chicken

Yields 4 servings

5 boneless, skinless chicken breast halves

2 (14 oz) jars salsa verde

¾ cup unsweetened coconut milk

1 yellow onion, sliced

3 cloves garlic, pressed

Note: This recipe uses 3 chicken breast halves—the extra 2 are to be used for Day Two's lunch.

Place chicken in a large slow cooker. Place remaining ingredients in a large bowl. Mix well, then pour mixture on top of chicken. Cook on low for 8–10 hours, until chicken is tender enough to shred with a fork. Remove the chicken from the slow cooker and place in a large bowl. Use two forks to shred the meat apart. Return chicken to the slow cooker, mix with salsa mixture, and serve.

Serving suggestion: Cauliflower "Rice" and a green salad

DAY TWO

Breakfast: Garden Morning Array

Yields 4 servings

8 hard-boiled eggs, peeled and halved, lengthwise

2 avocados, diced

3 vine-ripened tomatoes, diced

1 cucumber, sliced

1 cup strawberries (or seasonal fruit of your choice)

Sea salt and freshly ground black pepper to taste

This is a simple breakfast that is great for those busy mornings. You simply portion out each item onto everyone's plate, lightly season everything except the fruit with sea salt and freshly ground pepper, and you're done.

Lunch: Mexican Chicken Sliders

Yields 4 servings

16 whole lettuce leaves

1–2 cups leftover Tomatillo Shredded Chicken, heated (leftover from Day One's dinner)

2 vine-ripened tomatoes, sliced

1 avocado, sliced

1 red onion, sliced

1 handful cilantro, chopped fine

Salsa verde or your favorite salsa

Everyone should get two sliders in this recipe; your "buns" are the lettuce leaves. On top of a lettuce leaf, pile chicken, tomato, avocado, onion, cilantro, and a spoonful of your favorite salsa. Place another lettuce leaf on top and serve.

Dinner: Red Wine and Dine London Broil

Yields 4 servings

1 cup red wine

3 tablespoons apple cider vinegar

4 cloves garlic, pressed

1 teaspoon sea salt

1 teaspoon freshly ground black pepper

1 teaspoon dried rosemary

½ teaspoon onion powder

2 lbs London broil

In a large bowl, whisk together all ingredients except London broil. Place meat in a large zipper-style plastic bag, pour mixture inside, seal, and refrigerate for at least 4 hours or overnight. Before cooking, preheat grill to medium-high. Remove London broil from marinade and grill for 6–10 minutes per side, until cooked according to your preference (depending on thickness).

Serving suggestion: Mashed Faux-Tatoes and roasted asparagus

DAY THREE

Breakfast: Bacon Kale Scramble

Yields 4 servings

5 slices bacon

8 eggs

3 cloves garlic, pressed

½ yellow onion, chopped

1 cup chopped kale

1 teaspoon sea salt

1 teaspoon freshly ground black pepper

½ teaspoon crushed red pepper flakes

1 tablespoon ghee

Cook bacon; break into pieces.

Crack eggs into a large bowl and mix in remaining ingredients (including cooked bacon) except ghee. Whisk together and then heat ghee in a large skillet over medium-high heat. Pour mixture into pan and cook, stirring constantly, for 4–8 minutes or until eggs are cooked through.

Lunch: Paleo Egg Salad

Yields 4 servings

PALEO MAYO:

1 egg yolk

1 teaspoon Dijon mustard

1 teaspoon white wine vinegar

1 teaspoon sea salt

1 teaspoon garlic powder

1 teaspoon lemon juice

1 cup avocado oil (or olive oil)

EGG SALAD:

8 hard-boiled eggs, chopped or sliced

2 tablespoons Paleo mayo

1 tablespoon Dijon mustard

½ red onion, chopped

1 stalk celery, chopped

1 teaspoon sea salt

1 teaspoon paprika

1 teaspoon freshly ground black pepper

To make mayo: In a medium bowl, whisk together all ingredients except oil. Once the yolk begins to get slightly thickened and fluffy, gradually pour in oil, whisking frequently. Keep whisking for 2–5 minutes or until fully combined. Stir until you get the familiar mayonnaise consistency. (You will have plenty of leftover mayo to use in other recipes down the road.)

Egg salad: Place all ingredients in a large bowl, stir until fully mixed, and serve on large lettuce leaves.

Dinner: Cherry Pork

Yields 4 servings

- 1 cup pitted cherries (frozen is fine)
- 2 tablespoons apple cider vinegar
- 2 tablespoons red wine
- 2 cloves garlic, pressed
- 2 tablespoons raw honey
- 1 teaspoon sea salt
- 4 boneless pork chops
- 1 tablespoon ghee

In a food processor, combine all ingredients except pork and ghee; blend until smooth. Place pork in a large zipper-style bag. Pour mixture inside, seal, and marinate in refrigerator for at least 4 hours or overnight. Before cooking, heat ghee in a large skillet over medium-high heat. Remove pork from marinade and sear for 4–6 minutes per side or until cooked through.

Serving suggestion: Mashed Faux-Tatoes and sautéed bok choy and carrots

DAY FOUR

Breakfast: Canadian Bacon Roll-Ups

Yields 4 servings

- 6–8 eggs
- 12 slices Canadian bacon
- ½ red onion, chopped
- 1 handful cilantro, chopped fine
- Sea salt and freshly ground pepper to taste

Scramble eggs and season with salt and pepper. Heat another skillet over medium heat and quickly brown Canadian bacon (just 30 seconds to a minute per side).

Once bacon is browned, stuff each piece with eggs, onion, and cilantro. You can serve them like little breakfast tacos or burritos and use a toothpick to hold them together—a fun and easy breakfast your kids will love!

Lunch: Turkey Sprouts Wrap

Yields 4 servings

8 large slices cold-cut turkey
Dijon mustard
Paleo mayo
1 cucumber, sliced lengthwise
1 green bell pepper, sliced
1 cup sprouts of your choice

Lay out slices of turkey and spread a little Dijon and mayo on each slice, then layer the cucumber, bell pepper, and sprouts and roll the turkey up like you would a wrap. Serve 2 rolls per person.

Dinner: Lemon Roasted Chicken

4–6 lbs whole chicken
2 tablespoons ghee, melted
3 tablespoons lemon juice
1 teaspoon lemon zest
3 cloves garlic, pressed
1 teaspoon sea salt
1 teaspoon freshly ground black pepper
1 teaspoon dried rosemary

Preheat oven to 400 degrees. Place chicken in a large roasting pan and set aside. In a medium bowl, combine ghee, lemon juice, lemon zest, and garlic. Whisk together, then pour and rub all over chicken. Evenly season with salt, pepper, and rosemary, and place in the oven to roast for 1–1 ½ hours, or until cooked through. Keep leftovers for next day's lunch!

Serving suggestion: Roasted butternut squash and steamed broccoli

DAY FIVE

Breakfast: Mexican Egg Bake

Yields 4 servings

> 8 large eggs
> ½ red onion, chopped
> 1 green bell pepper, sliced
> 5 slices Canadian bacon, chopped
> 1 handful cilantro, chopped fine
> 1 teaspoon sea salt
> 1 teaspoon freshly ground black pepper
> 1 teaspoon cumin
> 1 tablespoon ghee, melted

Preheat oven to 375 degrees.

In a large bowl, crack eggs. Add remaining ingredients except ghee, and whisk together until well combined. Using a paper towel, spread melted ghee on all sides of a large casserole dish. Pour mixture into the dish and bake for 30–40 minutes or until the center is firm.

Lunch: Lemon Pepper Chicken Salad

Yields 4 servings

> 2 cups leftover Lemon Roasted Chicken, shredded or chopped
>   (from Day Four's dinner)
> 1 stalk celery, chopped

½ red onion, chopped

4 radishes, chopped

¼ cup unsweetened dried cranberries

2 tablespoons Paleo mayo

2 teaspoons Dijon mustard

1 ½ teaspoons lemon juice

1 teaspoon freshly ground black pepper

1 teaspoon sea salt

Place all ingredients in a large bowl and stir until combined. Serve.

Dinner: Sweet Lime Shrimp

Yields 4 servings

3 tablespoons raw honey

2 tablespoons lime juice

3 tablespoons white wine

2 tablespoons coconut oil, melted

3 cloves garlic, pressed

1 teaspoon sea salt

1 teaspoon freshly ground black pepper

½ teaspoon crushed red pepper flakes

2 lbs large shrimp, peeled and deveined

Wooden skewers (soak in water for 30 minutes so they won't catch fire)

Preheat outdoor grill to medium-high. In a large bowl, whisk together all ingredients except shrimp. Once ingredients are fully combined, throw shrimp in mixture and toss until all shrimp are coated. Skewer shrimp and grill for 3–5 minutes per side or until pink and opaque. Be sure to put aside leftovers for next day's lunch.

Serving suggestion: Cauliflower "Rice" and steamed green beans

DAY SIX

Breakfast: Cacao Banana Nut Smoothie

Yields 4 servings

8 scoops All-in-One Chai Smoothie Mix

2 frozen bananas

1–2 cups unsweetened almond milk

¼ cup almond butter

2 tablespoons cacao nibs

In a large blender, combine all ingredients (measure almond milk according to how thick you want your smoothie). Blend until smooth. It could take a few minutes to get almond butter and cacao nice and blended. Serve and enjoy.

Lunch: Shrimp Pico Tacos

Yields 4 servings

PICO DE GALLO:

2 vine-ripened tomatoes, chopped

½ yellow onion, chopped

2 cloves garlic, pressed

½ jalapeño, seeded and chopped (use a whole one if you like your food spicy)

1 handful cilantro, chopped

1 tablespoon lime juice

1 teaspoon sea salt

TACOS:

8 large lettuce leaves

2 cups shrimp, cooked (preferably leftovers from Day Five's dinner)

1 avocado, chopped

1 green bell pepper, chopped

In a food processor, place all pico de gallo ingredients. Pulse just to combine all ingredients, but don't puree (unless that's your preferred consistency). For the tacos, place shrimp in the lettuce, which will serve as your taco shells, and layer avocado and bell peppers on top. Add a scoop of pico de gallo, and serve.

Dinner: Spiced Turkey Meatballs

Yields 4 servings

1 ½ lbs ground turkey

2 tablespoons coconut oil, melted

1 egg

½ cup almond meal

1 yellow onion, chopped

3 cloves garlic, pressed

1 teaspoon sea salt

1 teaspoon paprika

1 teaspoon freshly ground black pepper

½ teaspoon cayenne pepper

½ teaspoon chili powder

½ teaspoon dried thyme

¼ teaspoon ground cumin

Preheat grill to medium-high. In a large bowl, combine all ingredients with your hands. Once ingredients are fully mixed, form 1–2-inch balls. Grill meatballs for 3–5 minutes per side, turning frequently, until cooked through (sometimes skewering helps when grilling them).

Serving suggestion: Cauliflower "Rice," baked sweet potato

DAY SEVEN

Breakfast: Blueberry Almond Pancakes

Yields 4 servings

  2 cups mashed bananas
  ½ cup blueberries
  ¼ cup almond meal
  1 egg
  2 tablespoons ghee, melted
  1 tablespoon vanilla extract
  1 tablespoon pure maple syrup
  1 teaspoon ground cinnamon
  1 tablespoon coconut oil
  ¼ cup chopped almonds
  2 tablespoons raw honey

In a medium bowl, combine bananas, blueberries, almond meal, egg, ghee, vanilla, maple syrup, and cinnamon until well blended, being sure to incorporate a great deal of air for a light batter. Melt the coconut oil in a large skillet over medium-low heat. Pour batter in ¼-cup portions into the skillet and cook until bubbles form in the middle of the pancakes. Flip carefully, and cook until just browned on each side, keeping an eye on them. Serve immediately, topped with chopped almonds and honey.

Lunch: Citrus Beef Salad

Yields 4 servings

  1 tablespoon ghee
  1 lb filet mignon, sliced into 1-inch strips
  2 cloves garlic, pressed

1 tablespoon paprika

1 tablespoon chopped jalapeño

6 cups baby spinach

¼ cup chopped green onion

½ cup shredded red cabbage

1 cup chopped orange

1 cup slivered almonds

2 tablespoons balsamic vinegar

Heat ghee in a skillet over medium heat. Add steak, garlic, and paprika, stirring often and browning the steak. Cook for 5–7 minutes, or until desired doneness.

In a large bowl, combine jalapeño, spinach, onion, cabbage, orange, almonds, and vinegar. Toss well to coat, and then divide among 4 plates. When steak is done, serve over the salad and enjoy.

Dinner: Spicy Clam Chowder

Yields 4 servings

2 tablespoons coconut oil

1 yellow onion, chopped

3 cloves garlic, minced

3 stalks celery, chopped

2 carrots, peeled and chopped

3 sweet potatoes, peeled and chopped

1 head cauliflower, chopped (approx. 5 cups)

6 cups low-sodium chicken broth

18 oz crabmeat

3 poblano peppers, roasted, skinned, seeded, and chopped

1 teaspoon sea salt

½ teaspoon freshly ground black pepper

1 teaspoon dried thyme

1 tablespoon arrowroot starch

2 tablespoons water

½ cup chopped parsley

6 slices bacon, cooked and crumbled

Melt the coconut oil in a large saucepan with a tight-fitting lid over medium-high heat. Add onion, garlic, celery, carrots, and sweet potatoes. Cook and stir until slightly tender. Add cauliflower and chicken broth; stir well to combine. Add crabmeat, poblano peppers, salt, pepper, and thyme. Bring mixture to a boil, then reduce heat to a simmer. In a small bowl or cup, combine arrowroot starch and water; add to soup mixture and continue to simmer until crabmeat is cooked, vegetables are tender, and chowder has thickened. Remove from heat. Top each serving with chopped parsley and crumbled bacon.

Serving suggestion: Large green salad with your choice of goodies

WEEK THREE SHOPPING LIST

Items marked with an asterisk (*) denote those needed for suggested side dishes and are, therefore, optional for the week's menu plan. Quantities will vary, depending on how often you choose to serve the suggested dish.

PROTEIN

- Eggs (28)
- Sausage links (8)
- Cold-cut turkey (½ lb)
- Bacon (12 slices)
- Canadian bacon (8 slices)
- Boneless, skinless chicken breast halves (20)
- Pork tenderloin (2 lbs)
- Halibut fillets, 6 oz (4)
- New York strip steaks (or cut of your choice), 6 oz (4)
- Sea scallops (1 lb)
- Canned tuna, 6 oz (3)

CONDIMENTS

- Coconut oil
- Raw honey
- Almond butter
- Ghee
- Olive oil
- Dijon mustard
- White wine vinegar
- Apple cider vinegar
- Balsamic vinegar

SPICES

- Sea salt
- Black peppercorns
- Ancho chili powder
- Paprika
- Unsweetened cocoa powder
- Ground ginger
- Garlic powder
- Cinnamon
- Onion powder
- Red pepper flakes

PRODUCE

- Radishes (4)
- Red onion (1)
- Sweet potatocs (2)
- Strawberries (1 cup)
- Cherry tomatoes (½ cup)
- Yellow onion (½)

- Green apples (5)
- Cucumbers (3)
- Green bell peppers (2)
- Red bell peppers (3)
- Yellow bell peppers (1)
- Garlic (10 cloves)
- Green onions (3)
- Spinach (9 cups)
- Romaine lettuce (2 cups)
- Lettuce leaves (8)
- Tomatoes (2)
- Avocados (6)
- Kale (4 cups)
- Lemons (2)
- Lime (1)
- Celery (2 stalks)
- Fresh basil (1 ½ cups)
- Salad greens* (your choice of dark greens—no iceberg lettuce!)
- Salad goodies* (whatever you like: slivered almonds, raisins, chopped onions, etc.)
- Cauliflower*
- Butternut squash*
- Kale*
- Swiss chard*
- Carrots*
- Cabbage*
- Asparagus*
- Broccoli*

CANNED GOODS

- Unsweetened coconut milk (in a carton, 3 cups + 3 tablespoons)
- Orange juice (½ cup)

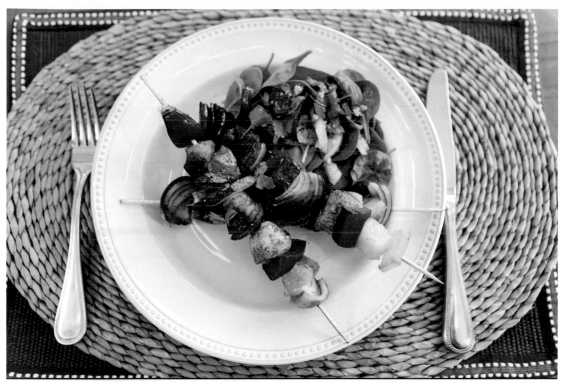

Sweet and Sour Chicken Pineapple Kebabs

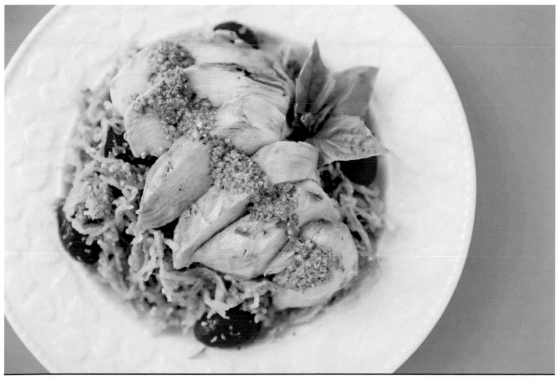

Pesto Chicken

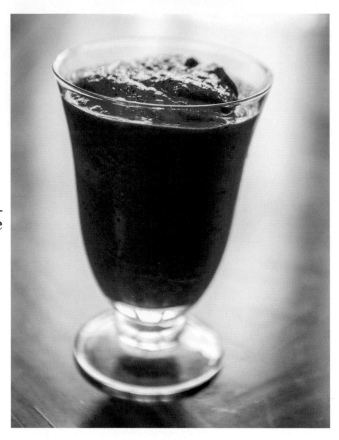

Paleo Power Smoothie

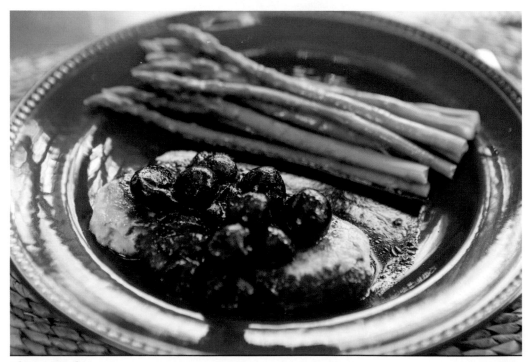

Cherry Pork

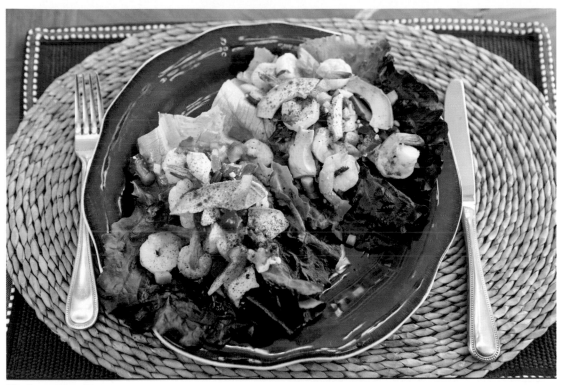

Shrimp Pico Tacos

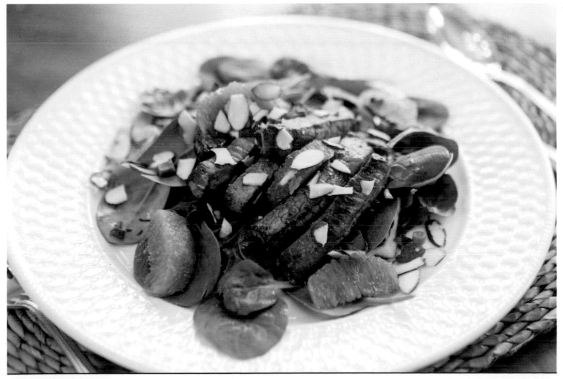

Citrus Beef Salad

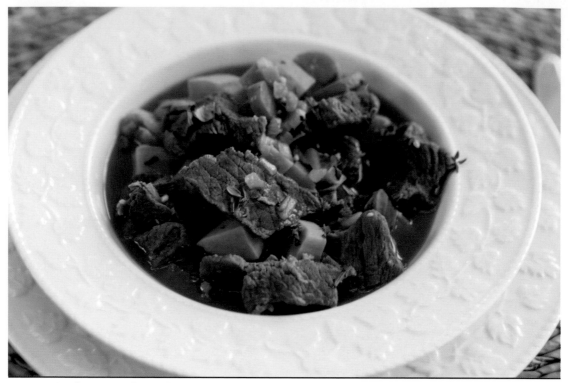

Savory Beef Stew with Herby Sweet Potatoes

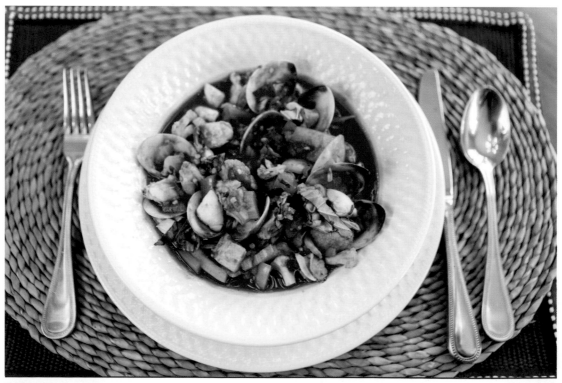

Paleo Cioppino

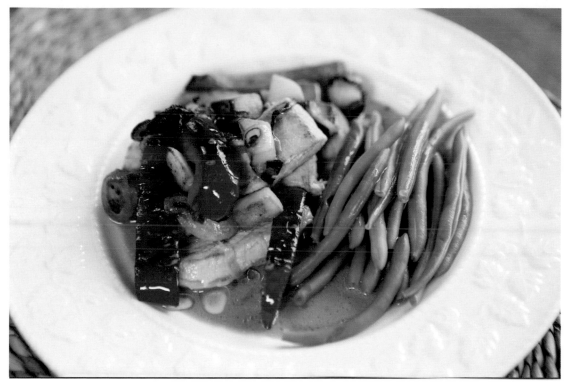

Pork and Apple Curry

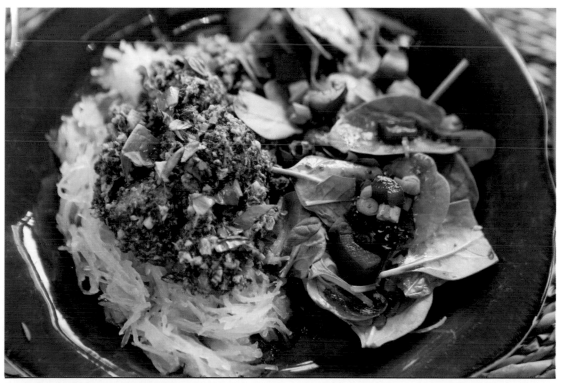

Sun-dried Tomato Meatballs with Pesto

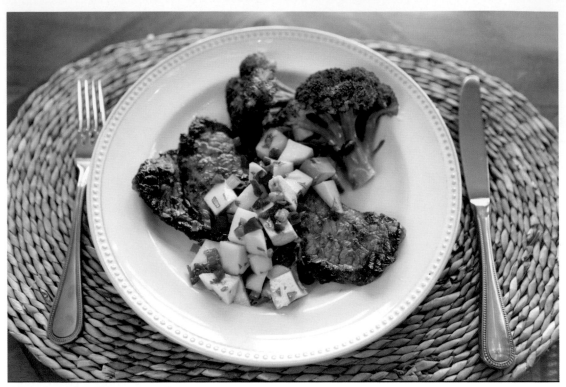

Ginger Beef and Mango Salsa

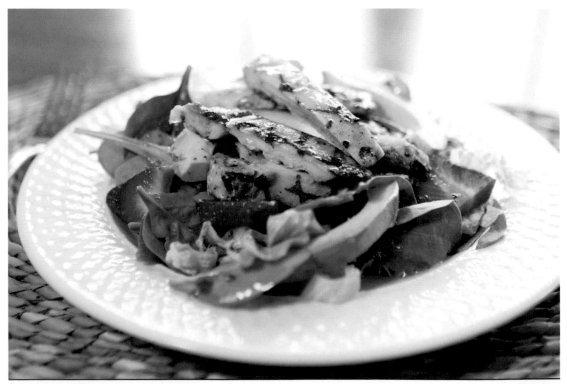

Chicken and Strawberry Salad

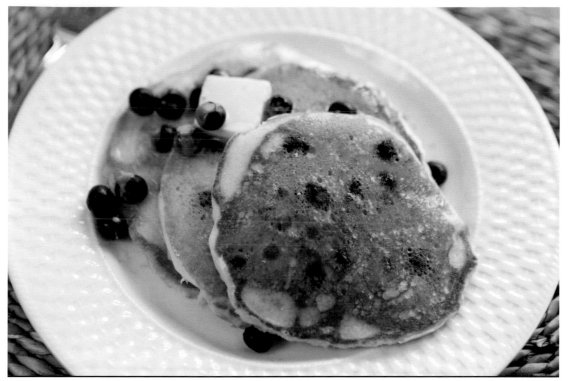

Blueberry Almond Pancakes

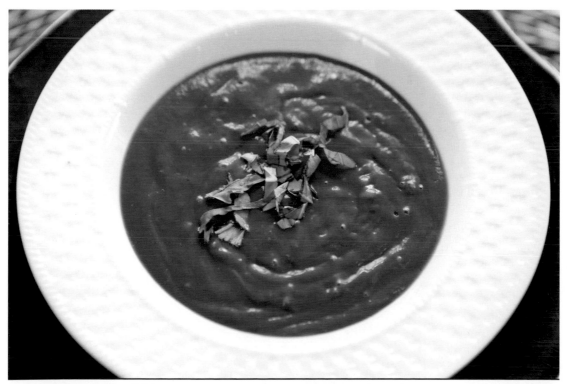

Roasted Tomato Basil Bisque

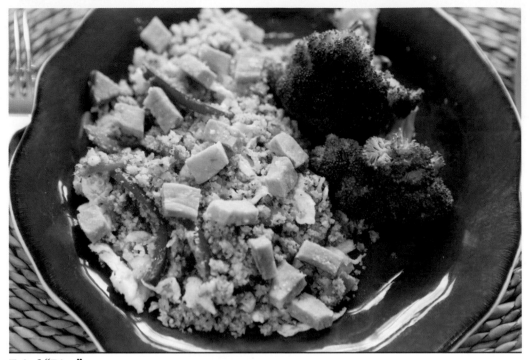

Fried "Rice"

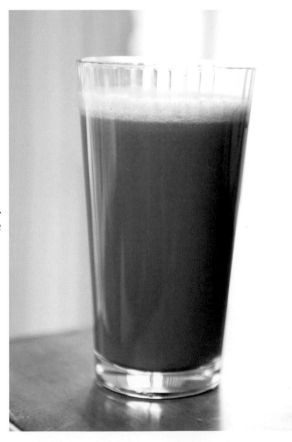

Super Green Juice

DRY GOODS

- Instant coffee (2 tablespoons)
- Roasted pecans (½ cup)
- Roasted pine nuts (2 tablespoons)
- Raw pine nuts (2 tablespoons)
- Raw walnuts (¼ cup)
- Unsweetened dried cranberries (¾ cup)
- All-in-One Vanilla Smoothie Mix (8 scoops, see Resources)
- All-in-One Chocolate Smoothie Mix (8 scoops)

DAIRY

- Butter

FREEZER

- Blackberries (1 cup)
- Bananas (2)
- Blueberries (½ cup)
- Strawberries (½ cup)
- Raspberries (½ cup)

OTHER

- Red wine
- Toothpicks

WEEK THREE RECIPES

DAY ONE

Breakfast: Easy as 1-2-3 Breakfast

Yields 4 servings

- 8 links sausage
- 1 ½ tablespoons coconut oil
- 3 cloves garlic, pressed
- 3 cups spinach
- 1 teaspoon sea salt
- 1 teaspoon freshly ground black pepper
- 8 eggs (cooked however you like—I usually do basted or scrambled with this recipe)

Cook sausage according to package directions. Heat coconut oil in a large skillet over medium-high heat. Add garlic, spinach, salt, and pepper. Sauté for 3–5 minutes or until spinach fully wilts. Serve with eggs and sausage.

Lunch: Lettuce Wraps

Yields 4 servings

WRAPS:

- 4 slices bacon
- Paleo mayo
- Dijon mustard
- 8 large lettuce leaves
- ½ lb cold-cut turkey (or cold-cut meat of your choice)
- 1 tomato, sliced

1 cucumber, sliced

4 radishes, sliced

1 avocado, sliced

LEMON VINAIGRETTE DIPPING SAUCE:

2 tablespoons lemon juice

2 tablespoons white wine vinegar

¼ cup olive oil

1 clove garlic, pressed

1 teaspoon sea salt

Cook bacon. When bacon slices have cooled, cut them in half.

Spread mayo and Dijon on the lettuce, then layer remaining ingredients and roll up like a wrap (you can use toothpicks to hold them together). In a medium bowl, whisk together ingredients for the dipping sauce and serve with wrap.

Dinner: Blackberry-Drizzled Chicken

Yields 4 servings

CHICKEN:

8 boneless, skinless chicken breast halves

Sea salt and freshly ground black pepper to taste

1 tablespoon coconut oil

BLACKBERRY SAUCE:

½ cup frozen blackberries

¼ cup red wine

2 tablespoons raw honey

1 teaspoon sea salt

1 tablespoon ghee

Note: This recipe uses 4 chicken breast halves—the extra 4 are to be used for Day Two's lunch. Try to save a couple of tablespoons of blackberry sauce as well.

Season chicken lightly with salt and pepper. Heat coconut oil in a large skillet and sear chicken for 4–6 minutes per side or until cooked through. Set aside.

In a food processor, blend blackberries, wine, honey, and salt. Heat ghee in a saucepan over medium-high heat and pour mixture into pan. Stir for about a minute, then reduce heat to medium and cover pan for another minute or two. Reduce heat to low and allow sauce to simmer for 8–10 minutes before serving over chicken.

Serving suggestion: Green salad (arugula would be good), roasted sweet potatoes

DAY TWO

Breakfast: Energizing Berry Smoothie

Yields 4 servings

8 scoops All-in-One Vanilla Smoothie Mix
½ cup frozen raspberries
½ cup frozen blueberries
½ cup frozen strawberries
½ cup frozen blackberries
1 frozen banana
10 ice cubes
1 cup unsweetened coconut milk

Place all ingredients in a blender and blend until smooth. Serve.

Lunch: Spinach Salad with Blackberry Vinaigrette

Yields 4 servings

SALAD:

4 cups spinach
½ red onion, sliced

1 green apple, chopped

½ cup chopped roasted pecans

¼ cup unsweetened dried cranberries

4 boneless, skinless chicken breast halves, cooked and chopped
   (leftover from Day One's dinner)

VINAIGRETTE:

2 tablespoons blackberry sauce from Blackberry-Drizzled Chicken recipe

2 tablespoons white wine vinegar

⅓ cup olive oil

1 teaspoon sea salt

Toss together all ingredients for the salad in a large serving bowl. In a medium bowl, whisk together ingredients for vinaigrette. Pour on salad, toss, and serve.

Dinner: Espresso-Rubbed Steak

Yields 4 servings

2 tablespoons extra-fine ground espresso (or instant coffee)

2 teaspoons ancho chili powder

1 teaspoon paprika

1 teaspoon sea salt

½ teaspoon ground ginger

1 tablespoon coconut oil, melted

4 (6 oz) New York strip steaks (or cut of your choice)

Preheat grill to medium-high. In a small bowl, whisk together dry ingredients. Brush coconut oil on all sides of each steak; rub dry mixture into steaks. Grill for 3–6 minutes per side or until cooked according to your preference.

Serving suggestion: Steamed Swiss chard, baked butternut squash

DAY THREE

Breakfast: Pepper Egg Bake

Yields 4 servings

- 2 green bell peppers
- 2 red bell peppers
- 2 tablespoons coconut oil, melted
- 8 eggs
- 1 teaspoon sea salt
- 1 teaspoon freshly ground black pepper
- 1 teaspoon paprika
- ½ teaspoon garlic powder
- ½ teaspoon onion powder

Preheat oven to 370 degrees. Prep bell peppers: Cut off stem, scoop out seeds, cut the smallest part of the bottom off, and cut in half horizontally (you should have 2 extra-large rings per pepper).

Grease an extra-large muffin pan with coconut oil. Then place bell pepper rings in muffin slots. Crack an egg into each ring. In a small bowl, combine remaining ingredients and evenly season the tops of each egg with the spices. Bake for 20–30 minutes or until eggs are cooked according to your preference.

Lunch: Tuna Salad

Yields 4 servings

- 3 (6 oz) cans tuna, drained
- 2 ½ tablespoons Paleo mayo
- 2 stalks celery, chopped
- ½ yellow onion, chopped

1 tablespoon lemon juice

1 teaspoon sea salt

1 teaspoon freshly ground black pepper

1 teaspoon garlic powder

Stir all ingredients in a large bowl until fully mixed. Serve in your favorite Part-Time Paleo method: on a lettuce leaf, atop a green salad, in an avocado half, or on cucumber slices.

Dinner: Orange Pepper Pork

Yields 4 servings

½ cup orange juice

3 tablespoons apple cider vinegar

1 red bell pepper, sliced

1 yellow bell pepper, sliced

1 teaspoon sea salt

1 teaspoon garlic powder

½ teaspoon onion powder

½ teaspoon crushed red pepper flakes

1–2 lbs pork tenderloin

1 tablespoon coconut oil, melted

In a bowl, mix together all ingredients except pork and oil. Place pork in a large slow cooker and pour oil over the top. Pour pepper mixture over the pork and cook on low for 8–10 hours. Save leftovers for Day Six's lunch.

Serving suggestion: Cauliflower "Rice" and steamed broccoli

DAY FOUR

Breakfast: Cocoa Avocado Smoothie

Yields 4 servings

    8 scoops All-in-One Chocolate Smoothie Mix

    2 avocados, pitted and peeled

    1 frozen banana

    1 cup unsweetened coconut milk

    6 ice cubes

    3 tablespoons raw honey

    1 tablespoon unsweetened cocoa powder

Combine all ingredients in blender. Blend until smooth and serve.

Lunch: Cucumber Chicken Sandwiches

Yields 4 servings

    3 boneless, skinless chicken breast halves

    1–2 cucumbers, sliced

    Paleo mayo

    Dijon mustard

    1 tomato, sliced

    ½ red onion, sliced

Roast chicken breast halves and slice after they've rested for at least 5 minutes.

    Use cucumber slices as "bread" and spread mayo and mustard on each slice. Stack chicken, tomato, and onion between two cucumber slices, and serve your mini-sandwiches.

Dinner: Coconut Lime Chicken

Yields 4 servings

    3 tablespoons unsweetened coconut milk

    2 tablespoons lime juice

    1 teaspoon lime zest

    1 teaspoon sea salt

    1 teaspoon freshly ground black pepper

    1 teaspoon garlic powder

    ½ teaspoon paprika

    ½ teaspoon chili powder

    ½ teaspoon cayenne pepper

    ½ teaspoon onion powder

    5 boneless, skinless chicken breast halves

    1 tablespoon coconut oil

Note: This recipe uses 4 chicken breast halves—the extra are to be used for Day Five's lunch.

In a medium bowl, whisk together coconut milk and lime juice. In a small bowl, mix together zest and spices. Dip each chicken breast half into the coconut lime juice mixture, and season evenly on all sides with dry mix. Heat coconut oil in a large skillet over medium-high heat and sear chicken for 4–6 minutes per side or until cooked through.

Serving suggestion: Cauliflower "Rice" and sautéed cabbage and grated carrots

DAY FIVE

Breakfast: Almond-Dipped Cinnamon Apples

Yields 4 servings

⅓ cup almond butter
2 tablespoons raw honey
4 green apples, sliced
Cinnamon

In a medium bowl, whisk together almond butter and honey, and set aside. Dust apples lightly with cinnamon and serve with almond-honey dip!

Lunch: Chicken and Strawberry Salad

Yields 4 servings

2 cups spinach
2 cups romaine lettuce
1 cup chopped strawberries
1 cup leftover cooked Coconut Lime Chicken (from Day Four's dinner)
¼ cup chopped raw walnuts
1 avocado, chopped
3–4 tablespoons Leanne's Basic Vinaigrette (recipe on page 95)

Place all ingredients in a large bowl. Toss until fully mixed together. Serve.

Dinner: Bacon-Wrapped Scallops

Yields 4 servings

1 lb fresh sea scallops
8 slices peppered bacon, cut in half

through. Season lightly with salt and pepper. Reserve half of the chicken for Day Seven's Warm Kale Salad. In a big bowl, scoop squash from the shell, add chicken and pesto, toss, and serve!

Serving suggestion: Roasted asparagus

DAY SEVEN

Breakfast: Avocado Egg Bakes

Yields 4 servings

2 avocados, halved (do not peel)
4 eggs
Sea salt and freshly ground black pepper to taste
½ teaspoon cayenne pepper
½ teaspoon chili powder
½ teaspoon garlic powder

Preheat oven to 350 degrees. Place avocados in a small baking dish, crack an egg into each half, season with spices, and bake for 20 minutes or until eggs are cooked through.

Lunch: Warm Kale Salad

Yields 4 servings

1 tablespoon coconut oil
4 cups kale, chopped
3 cloves garlic, pressed
1 teaspoon sea salt
2 tablespoons roasted pine nuts
½ cup halved cherry tomatoes

2 cups leftover Pesto Chicken, chopped

⅓ cup unsweetened dried cranberries

3–4 tablespoons Leanne's Basic Vinaigrette (recipe on page 95)

Heat coconut oil in a large skillet over medium-high heat and add kale, garlic, and salt. Sauté for 3–5 minutes, until kale wilts, then transfer kale to a large bowl, toss with remaining ingredients, and serve.

Dinner: Baja Halibut

Yields 4 servings

1 teaspoon sea salt

1 teaspoon freshly ground black pepper

1 teaspoon paprika

½ teaspoon cayenne pepper

½ teaspoon chili powder

½ teaspoon garlic powder

½ teaspoon ground cumin

¼ teaspoon onion powder

4 (6 oz) halibut fillets

1 tablespoon coconut oil

In a small bowl, combine all spices. Season fillets evenly with dry spices. Heat coconut oil in a large skillet over medium-high heat and sear each fillet for 2–4 minutes per side or until cooked through.

Serving suggestion: Large green salad and roasted beets

WEEK FOUR SHOPPING LIST

Items marked with an asterisk (*) denote those needed for suggested side dishes and are, therefore, optional for the week's menu plan.

Quantities will vary, depending on how often you choose to serve the suggested dish.

PROTEIN

- Eggs (29)
- Bacon (14 strips)
- Boneless, skinless chicken breast halves (6)
- Chicken sausage links (5 large)
- Flank steak (3 lbs)
- Cold-cut turkey breast (½ lb)
- Cold-cut ham (½ lb)
- Ground turkey (2 lbs)
- Andouille sausage (5 oz)
- Pork tenderloin (2 lbs)
- Lamb chops (6–8)
- Canned tuna, 6 oz (3)
- Peeled and deveined shrimp (2 lbs)
- Salmon fillets, 6 oz (4)

CONDIMENTS

- Coconut oil
- Raw honey
- Ghee
- Olive oil
- Dijon mustard
- Balsamic vinegar
- Apple cider vinegar
- Coconut aminos (see Resources)
- Salsa
- Almond butter

SPICES

- Sea salt
- Black peppercorns
- Red pepper flakes
- Cayenne pepper
- Dried sage
- Paprika
- Dried thyme
- Bay leaf
- Garlic powder
- Onion powder
- Cumin

PRODUCE

- Radishes (4)
- Red onions (2 ½)
- Yellow onions (3, plus extra for serving suggestion)
- Apple (1)
- Green bell pepper (1)
- Zucchini (2 large)
- Garlic (28 cloves)
- Spinach (3 cups)
- Tomatoes (3)
- Romaine lettuce leaves (24 large)
- Kale (1 cup, plus extra for serving suggestion)
- Avocado (1)
- Mushrooms (1 cup)
- Lemon (1)
- Limes (2)
- Banana (1)
- Strawberries (½ cup)

- Celery (3 stalks)
- Fresh mint (⅓ cup)
- Spaghetti squash
- Bok choy
- Swiss chard
- Salad greens* (your choice of dark greens—no iceberg lettuce!)
- Salad goodies* (whatever you like: slivered almonds, raisins, chopped onions, etc.)
- Cauliflower*
- Broccoli*
- Asparagus*
- Green beans*

CANNED GOODS

- Unsweetened coconut milk (in a carton, 2 ½ cups)
- Unsweetened almond milk (1 ½ cups)
- Diced tomatoes (2 14-oz cans)
- Low-sodium chicken broth (4 cups)

DRY GOODS

- All-in-One Vanilla Smoothie Mix (16 scoops, see Resources)
- All-in-One Chai Smoothie Mix (8 scoops)
- Raisins (¼ cup)
- Almond meal (⅓ cup)
- Unsweetened shredded coconut (⅔ cup)
- Sun-dried tomatoes, not packed in oil (4)

FREEZER

- Peaches (2 cups)
- Pineapple (½ cup)
- Bananas (2)

• Muffin liners

WEEK FOUR RECIPES

DAY ONE

Breakfast: Kale 'n' Eggs

Yields 4 servings

    5 large links chicken sausage
    1 tablespoon coconut oil
    2 cloves garlic, pressed
    ½ yellow onion, chopped
    1 cup chopped kale
    8 eggs, whisked together in a bowl
    1 teaspoon sea salt
    1 teaspoon freshly ground black pepper

Note: This recipe uses 2 sausage links—the extra are to be used for lunch.

Cook sausage. Chop when cooled.

Heat coconut oil in a large skillet over medium-high heat. Add garlic and onion, and sauté for 3–5 minutes. While that's cooking, mix kale into beaten eggs. Pour mixture into skillet, stirring constantly, and add salt and pepper. Cook for 6–8 minutes or until cooked through.

Lunch: Baked Stuffed Zucchini

Yields 4 servings

    2 large zucchini, halved lengthwise and seeded
    3 large links chicken sausage, cooked and chopped (leftover from breakfast)
    ½ yellow onion, chopped
    2 cloves garlic, pressed

Preheat oven to 350 degrees.

Place zucchini halves in a small baking pan and stuff with sausage, onion, and garlic. Bake for 20–30 minutes and serve.

Dinner: Asian Grilled Chicken

Yields 4 servings

    3 cloves garlic, pressed
    3 tablespoons coconut aminos
    1 teaspoon sea salt
    1 tablespoon raw honey
    6 boneless, skinless chicken breast halves
    1 tablespoon coconut oil

Note: This recipe uses 4 chicken breast halves—the extra 2 are for Day Four's lunch.

In a medium bowl, whisk together all ingredients except chicken and coconut oil. Place chicken in the bowl with the mixture, making sure all pieces are fully saturated. Heat coconut oil in a large skillet over medium-high heat. Sear chicken for 4–6 minutes per side or until cooked through.

Serving suggestion: Cauliflower "Rice" and a big green salad

DAY TWO

Breakfast: Coconut Peach Smoothie

Yields 4 servings

> 8 scoops All-in-One Chai Smoothie Mix
>
> 2 cups frozen peaches
>
> 1 banana
>
> 10 ice cubes
>
> 1 ½ cups unsweetened coconut milk
>
> 1 tablespoon coconut oil

Place all ingredients in a blender and blend until smooth. Serve.

Lunch: Paleo BLT Stacks

Yields 4 servings

> 8 strips bacon
>
> 8 large romaine leaves
>
> Paleo mayo
>
> Dijon mustard
>
> 1 tomato, sliced
>
> ½ lb cold-cut turkey breast

Cook bacon. On top of each piece of lettuce, spread the mayo and mustard; layer remaining ingredients to form stacks.

Dinner: Sun-dried Tomato Flank Steak

Yields 4 servings

    4 sun-dried tomatoes, chopped
    3 tablespoons balsamic vinegar
    2 tablespoons olive oil
    3 cloves garlic, pressed
    1 teaspoon sea salt
    1 teaspoon freshly ground black pepper
    3 lbs flank steak

In a food processor, combine all ingredients except steak. Blend until smooth. Place steak in a large zipper-style plastic bag. Pour mixture inside and seal. Marinate in refrigerator for 4 hours or overnight. Before cooking, preheat grill to medium-high. Remove steak from marinade and grill for 6–10 minutes per side or until according to your preference. Reserve leftovers for Day Three's lunch.

    Serving suggestion: Roasted green beans and Mashed Faux-Tatoes

DAY THREE

Breakfast: Tropical Spinach Smoothie

Yields 4 servings

    1 cup spinach
    ½ cup frozen pineapple
    1 tablespoon coconut oil
    ½ cup strawberries
    8 scoops All-in-One Vanilla Smoothie Mix
    1 cup unsweetened coconut milk
    10 ice cubes

Combine all ingredients in blender and blend until smooth.

Lunch: Tacos de Carne

Yields 4 servings

    8 large romaine lettuce leaves

    2 cups leftover Sun-dried Tomato Flank Steak, heated and sliced

    1 tomato, chopped

    ½ red onion, chopped

    1 avocado, chopped

    Salsa

    1 lime, cut into wedges

Fill each lettuce leaf with steak, tomato, onion, avocado, and a scoop of salsa. Serve with a wedge of lime.

Dinner: Simple Caliente Pork

Yields 4 servings

    ⅓ cup apple cider vinegar

    1 teaspoon sea salt

    1 teaspoon crushed red pepper flakes

    1 red onion, chopped

    4 cloves garlic, pressed

    1–2 lbs pork tenderloin

    1 tablespoon coconut oil, melted

In a bowl, mix together all ingredients except pork and oil. Place pork in a large slow cooker and pour oil over the top. Pour mixture over the top of the pork and cook on low for 8–10 hours, until tender enough to shred. Reserve leftovers for Day Four's breakfast.

    Serving suggestion: Mashed Faux-Tatoes and steamed broccoli

DAY FOUR

Breakfast: Mexican Pork Frittata

Yields 4 servings

- 8 eggs
- 1 overflowing cup of leftover Simple Caliente Pork
- 1 cup spinach
- 2 cloves garlic, pressed
- 1 teaspoon sea salt
- 1 teaspoon freshly ground black pepper
- ½ tablespoon coconut oil, melted

Preheat oven to 375 degrees. Beat eggs in a medium-size bowl, and add remaining ingredients except coconut oil. Grease a 10-inch baking dish with the coconut oil, pour in mixture, and bake for 30–40 minutes or until cooked through.

Lunch: Apple Chicken Salad

Yields 4 servings

- 2 chicken breast halves, cooked and chopped (leftover from Day One's dinner)
- 3 tablespoons Paleo mayo
- 1 large apple, chopped
- ½ red onion, chopped
- 1 stalk celery, chopped
- ¼ cup unsweetened raisins

In a large bowl, mix together all ingredients. Serve.

Dinner: Garlic Mint Lamb

Yields 4 servings

⅓ cup fresh mint

3 cloves garlic

1 tablespoon apple cider vinegar

1 teaspoon sea salt

1 teaspoon freshly ground black pepper

½ teaspoon onion powder

1 tablespoon coconut oil, melted

6–8 lamb chops

Preheat grill to medium-high. Combine all ingredients except lamb in a food processor. Rub lamb with mixture and grill for 4–6 minutes per side or until cooked through.

Serving suggestion: Mashed Faux-Tatoes and steamed green beans

DAY FIVE

Breakfast: Mushroom Quiche Muffins

Yields 4 servings

6 strips bacon

1 cup chopped mushrooms

1 cup chopped fresh spinach

3 cloves garlic, pressed

2 tablespoons coconut oil, melted

1 teaspoon sea salt

1 teaspoon ground cumin

1 teaspoon freshly ground black pepper

8 eggs, beaten

Muffin liners

Preheat oven to 350 degrees. Cook bacon, and chop once cooled. Add all ingredients to the bowl of beaten eggs, and whisk together. Line a muffin tin with paper liners, and fill each cup halfway with egg mixture. Bake for 20–30 minutes or until cooked through.

Lunch: Radish Tuna Salad

Yields 4 servings

- 3 (6 oz) cans tuna, drained
- 3 tablespoons Paleo mayo
- 1 teaspoon sea salt
- 1 stalk celery, chopped
- 4 radishes, chopped
- 1 tablespoon lemon juice
- 1 teaspoon freshly ground black pepper
- 1 teaspoon garlic powder

Place all ingredients in a large bowl and stir until fully combined. Serve.

Dinner: Honey Coconut Shrimp

Yields 4 servings

- 2 lbs shrimp, peeled and deveined
- 1 teaspoon sea salt
- 1 teaspoon crushed red pepper flakes
- 2 tablespoons raw honey
- ⅓ cup unsweetened shredded coconut
- 2 tablespoons ghee

Note: This recipe uses 1 ½ lbs shrimp—the extra ½ lb is to be used in Day Six's lunch.

Season shrimp with salt and red pepper flakes. Drizzle honey on all sides of shrimp. Roll shrimp in coconut to cover. Heat ghee in a large skillet over medium-high heat and sear shrimp for 3–5 minutes per side or until pink and opaque.

Serving suggestion: Cauliflower "Rice" and sautéed bok choy and onions

DAY SIX

Breakfast: Almond Banana Power Smoothie

Yields 4 servings

 2 frozen bananas
 ¼ cup almond butter
 1 ½ cups unsweetened almond milk
 8 scoops All-in-One Vanilla Smoothie Mix
 10 ice cubes
 1 tablespoon raw honey

Place all ingredients in blender and blend until smooth.

Lunch: Coconut Shrimp Gumbo

Yields 4 servings

 1 tablespoon coconut oil
 1 yellow onion, diced
 3 cloves garlic, pressed
 1 stalk celery, diced
 ½ cup diced green bell pepper
 2 (14 oz) cans diced tomatoes
 4 cups chicken broth
 1 cup cooked, chopped Andouille sausage
 1 bay leaf

2 teaspoons sea salt

1 teaspoon freshly ground black pepper

½ teaspoon cayenne pepper

½ teaspoon dried thyme

1 cup leftover Honey Coconut Shrimp

Heat coconut oil in a large pot and add onion, garlic, celery, and bell pepper. Stir and cook for 5 minutes, then add remaining ingredients. Stir well, reduce heat to low, and cover pot. Simmer for 20 minutes, stirring occasionally, and serve.

Dinner: Turkey Meatloaf

Yields 4 servings

2 lbs ground turkey

1 egg, beaten

⅓ cup almond meal

3 tablespoons coconut aminos

1 yellow onion, chopped

3 cloves garlic, pressed

1 teaspoon sea salt

1 teaspoon freshly ground black pepper

1 teaspoon paprika

½ teaspoon cayenne pepper

½ teaspoon dried sage

1 tablespoon coconut oil, melted

Preheat oven to 375 degrees. In a large bowl, combine all ingredients, except oil, with your hands. Grease a loaf pan with melted oil, place mixture in pan, and bake for 1 hour or until cooked through, reaching an internal temperature of 165 degrees. Save leftovers for Day Seven's breakfast.

Serving suggestion: Mashed Faux-Tatoes and steamed kale

DAY SEVEN

Breakfast: Meatloaf Fried Eggs

Yields 4 servings

4 large slices Turkey Meatloaf
1 tablespoon coconut oil
4 eggs
Sea salt and freshly ground black pepper to taste

Use a small round cookie cutter to make a hole in the center of each meatloaf slice. Heat coconut oil in a large skillet over medium-high heat. Place meatloaf carefully in skillet, then crack an egg into the center of each slice. Season egg with salt and pepper. After 1–2 minutes (or when egg whites start to solidify), very carefully flip the meatloaf with the egg and cook another 1–2 minutes before serving.

Lunch: Ham and Mustard Wrap

Yields 4 servings

Paleo mayo
Dijon mustard
8 large romaine lettuce leaves
½ lb cold-cut ham
1 tomato, sliced
½ red onion, sliced

Spread mayo and mustard onto lettuce leaves, then layer remaining ingredients and roll up like a wrap. Serve.

Dinner: Honey-Glazed Salmon

Yields 4 servings

SALMON:

1 teaspoon sea salt

1 teaspoon freshly ground black pepper

1 teaspoon paprika

½ teaspoon cayenne pepper

4 (6 oz) salmon fillets

1 tablespoon coconut oil

HONEY GLAZE:

3 tablespoons raw honey

1 tablespoon ghee

In a small bowl, combine all spices. Season fillets evenly with spice mix. Heat coconut oil in a large skillet over medium-high heat and sear each fillet for 2–4 minutes per side or until cooked through.

In the same pan, over medium heat, whisk together honey and ghee. Reduce heat to medium-low and allow to simmer for 4 minutes, or until it reaches a shiny glaze consistency. Serve over salmon.

Serving suggestion: Large green salad and steamed Swiss chard

8

CHAPTER EIGHT

A FEW STEWS AND OTHER SLOW COOKER MAGIC

O ne of the best appliances for cooking in the Part-Time Paleo life-style is the magical slow cooker. Some people call it a Crock-Pot (Rival owns the brand, by the way); some call it a slow cooker. At home, I call it a "crock cooker"—a hybridization that you're welcome to use for this beloved appliance with my compliments.

Whatever you call these mighty small appliances, they do make life a lot easier. Remember, there are many brands of the slow-cookin', crock-lovin' contraption. Some cook hotter than others, some are older and slower, some are newer and faster, and depending on how full they are, the cooking instructions can be a guide, not a definitive final word—your mileage may vary.

Slow cookers are fabulous for Paleoistas because they take so much work out of meal prep and because they are ideal for extract-ing minerals and nutrients from all those bones you're going to be con-suming.

Because slow cookers aren't just for soups and bone broth, I just had to put together a few of my favorite easy slow-cookin' recipes for you. I know you're going to love them as much my family does—enjoy!

PALEO SLOW COOKER RECIPES

Middle Eastern Pork and Sweet Potato Stew

Yields 6 servings

- 2 ½ lbs pork tenderloin, cubed
- 1 teaspoon sea salt
- 1 teaspoon freshly ground black pepper
- ½ teaspoon ground cumin
- ½ teaspoon ground coriander
- 3 shallots, peeled and sliced
- 2 cloves garlic, pressed
- 1 poblano pepper, chopped
- 1 medium yellow bell pepper, chopped
- 1 medium red bell pepper, chopped
- 1 medium tomato, diced
- 2 medium sweet potatoes, peeled and diced
- 2 mangoes, peeled and chopped
- 4 cups low-sodium chicken broth
- Juice of half a lime
- 2 tablespoons chopped fresh thyme

Place stew meat in a large bowl; sprinkle with seasonings. With your hands, thoroughly rub seasonings into the meat. Place next 8 ingredients in slow cooker, add seasoned pork, and pour broth and lime juice over the top. Stir mixture to blend well. Cover and cook on low for 5–6 hours or until pork and vegetables are tender (the mangoes will break down and become part of the cooking juices). Stir in chopped thyme and serve.

Serving suggestion: Baby spinach salad

PART-TIME PALEO FIX

Switch out sweet potatoes for organic white potatoes or, even better, purple potatoes.

Chicken Stew with Fall Veggies

Yields 6 servings

3 lbs boneless chicken thighs, cubed

1 tablespoon sea salt

1 teaspoon freshly ground black pepper

2 cloves garlic, minced

6 sprigs thyme

4 medium stalks celery, chopped

1 medium red onion, chopped

2 cups acorn squash, cubed

1 bulb fennel, cored and sliced

6 cremini (baby portobello) mushrooms, sliced

4 cups low-sodium chicken broth

1 tablespoon tomato paste

1 tablespoon lemon juice

2 tablespoons chopped rosemary

Place chicken in a large bowl; toss with salt, pepper, and garlic. Place thyme and vegetables in slow cooker. In a medium bowl, whisk together broth, tomato paste, and lemon juice until well combined. Pour mixture into slow cooker, then add seasoned chicken and stir to blend well. Cover and cook on low for 5–6 hours or until chicken is fork-tender and vegetables are cooked through. Before serving, stir in chopped rosemary.

Serving suggestion: Apple, walnut, and arugula salad with balsamic vinegar

Cream of Chicken Stew

Yields 6 servings

6 (6 oz) boneless, skinless chicken thighs

2 teaspoons sea salt, divided

1 teaspoon ground white pepper, divided

1 teaspoon dried thyme

1 teaspoon dried rosemary

1 medium yellow onion, chopped

½ lb cremini (baby portobello) mushrooms, sliced

3 medium stalks celery, chopped

2 medium parsnips, peeled and chopped

2 cups full-fat unsweetened canned coconut milk

1 teaspoon Dijon mustard

1 teaspoon lemon juice

Place chicken in a large bowl; sprinkle with half of the salt, half of the white pepper, the thyme and rosemary, and the onion. With your hands, thoroughly rub this mixture into the chicken; set aside. Place mushrooms, celery, and parsnips in slow cooker. In a small bowl, whisk together coconut milk, mustard, and lemon juice along with remaining salt and pepper. Pour mixture over vegetables in slow cooker, then add chicken. Stir to blend well. Cover and cook on low for 4–5 hours or until chicken is cooked through and vegetables are tender.

Serving suggestion: Sautéed dandelion greens with bacon and onion

---

Seafood Creole Stew

Yields 8 servings

2 medium green bell peppers, chopped

2 medium stalks celery, chopped

1 jalapeño, sliced

2 (14.5 oz) cans diced tomatoes

1 cup tomato sauce

1 teaspoon chili powder

1 teaspoon sea salt

1 teaspoon ground white pepper

1 tablespoon raw honey

1 lb medium shrimp, peeled and deveined

½ lb mahimahi, cubed

Place all ingredients, except for the shrimp and mahimahi, in the slow cooker. Cover and cook on high for 2–3 hours. Add shrimp and mahimahi for 30 minutes before serving, until shrimp are pink and opaque and the fish is cooked through.

Serving suggestion: Cauliflower "Rice" and sautéed Swiss chard

Braised Beef and Squash

Yields 6 servings

6 beef shanks
1 teaspoon sea salt
½ teaspoon ground cumin
½ teaspoon ground cinnamon
½ teaspoon ground allspice
½ teaspoon freshly ground black pepper
6 cloves garlic, pressed
3 cups low-sodium chicken broth
½ cup canned tomatoes in sauce
½ cup chopped celery
1 butternut squash, peeled and cubed
1 lemon, zest and juice
1 tablespoon chopped basil

Place beef shanks in a large bowl; sprinkle with dry seasonings. With your hands, thoroughly rub the spices mixture into the beef shanks. Place shanks in the slow cooker. Add next 6 ingredients; stir to blend well. Cover and cook on low for 8–10 hours or until shanks are falling off the bone. Garnish with chopped basil and serve.

Serving suggestion: Steamed broccoli

Citrus and Spice Lamb Tagine

Yields 6 servings

  4 lbs extra-lean lamb roast, cubed
  ½ teaspoon crushed red pepper flakes
  ½ tablespoon ground cumin
  ½ teaspoon sea salt
  ½ teaspoon freshly ground black pepper
  3 cloves garlic, pressed
  4 medium purple (or orange) carrots, chopped
  2 medium parsnips, peeled and diced
  6 roma tomatoes, chopped
  1 lime, juice and zest
  1 cup red wine vinegar
  3 cups low-sodium beef broth
  ¼ cup slivered almonds, toasted
  ¼ cup dried apricots
  ½ cup chopped mint

In a large bowl, place first 6 ingredients. Thoroughly rub the seasonings into the meat. In a slow cooker, place carrots and parsnips along with tomatoes, lime juice and zest, vinegar, and broth. Add lamb and stir well to blend ingredients. Add almonds and dried apricots. Cook on low for 6–7 hours or until lamb is fork-tender. Before serving, stir in the chopped mint and serve.

   Serving suggestion: Roasted acorn squash and steamed brussels sprouts

Savory Beef Stew with Herby Sweet Potatoes

Yields 6 servings

  4 lbs beef stew meat, cubed
  1 tablespoon sea salt
  ½ tablespoon freshly ground black pepper

2 cloves garlic, minced

1 medium yellow onion, sliced

1 (14.5 oz) can diced tomatoes

3 medium sweet potatoes, peeled and diced

4 stalks celery, chopped

1 medium carrot, chopped

½ cup sliced dried apricots

¼ cup chopped fresh thyme

¼ cup chopped fresh rosemary

1 tablespoon cider vinegar

3 cups low-sodium beef broth

2 tablespoons chopped fresh sage

Place beef in a large bowl. Add salt, pepper, and garlic, and toss well. Place sliced onion in slow cooker. Top with beef mixture, then add remaining ingredients except sage. Cover and cook on low for 6–7 hours or until beef is fork-tender and cooked through. Stir in chopped sage and serve.

Serving suggestion: A big spinach salad

Paleo Cioppino

Yields 10 servings (Yay! Leftovers!)

1 tablespoon coconut oil

1 cup diced white onion

1 cup diced green bell pepper

1 cup diced red bell pepper

½ cup sliced green onions

1 fennel bulb, cored and sliced

6 plum (roma) tomatoes, diced

2 cups chopped cauliflower (approximately half a medium-size cauliflower)

4 cloves garlic, minced

2 cups tomato sauce

1 cup low-sodium chicken broth

1 bay leaf

3 tablespoons chopped basil leaves

1 teaspoon freshly ground black pepper

1 teaspoon sea salt

20 littleneck clams, scrubbed clean

1 lb cod, cubed

8 oz crabmeat

20 medium shrimp, peeled and deveined

Combine all ingredients except clams, shrimp, cod, and crabmeat in a slow cooker. Cover and cook on low for 3 hours. Add all seafood except shrimp one hour before serving; add shrimp ½ hour before serving. Serve and enjoy.

Serving suggestion: Arugula salad with walnuts and apples

Coconut Chicken and Broccoli Stew

Yields 6 servings

2 tablespoons coconut oil

1 medium white onion, chopped

3 lbs boneless, skinless chicken breast halves, cubed

1 teaspoon sea salt

1 ½ tablespoons sweet curry powder

1 teaspoon ground ginger

1 teaspoon ground cinnamon

3 cups chopped broccoli

1 cup raisins

2 green apples, diced

1 (14 oz) can unsweetened coconut milk

2 cups low-sodium chicken broth

1 lime, juiced

1 cup unsweetened coconut cream

½ cup unsweetened toasted coconut flakes

In a sauté pan, melt the coconut oil over medium-high heat. Add chopped onion and sauté until golden, then transfer to a blender or food processor. Cool slightly, then puree until liquefied. Place cubed chicken in slow cooker. Sprinkle with salt, curry powder, ginger, and cinnamon, then thoroughly rub seasonings into the meat. Add onion puree along with remaining ingredients and stir to blend well. Cover and cook on low for 7–8 hours or until chicken is fork-tender. Serve with a sprinkle of toasted coconut.

Serving suggestion: Whipped and buttery organic purple potatoes (It wouldn't hurt to throw in a little kale salad, too.)

Braised Pork Roast with Cuban Vegetables

Yields 6 servings

3 lbs boneless pork tenderloin, cubed

1 teaspoon sea salt

1 teaspoon freshly ground black pepper

2 cloves garlic, minced

1 medium red bell pepper, chopped

1 medium green bell pepper, chopped

1 medium red onion, sliced

3 medium sweet potatoes, peeled and diced

2 tablespoons Dijon mustard

1 tablespoon honey

4 plum (roma) tomatoes, diced

1 (28 oz) can diced tomatoes

1 cup low-sodium chicken broth

½ teaspoon crushed red pepper flakes

½ teaspoon dried sage

Place pork in slow cooker. Rub well with salt, pepper, and garlic. Add remaining ingredients. Cover and cook on low for 5–6 hours or until pork is cooked through and vegetables are tender. Serve and enjoy.

9

CHAPTER NINE

FROZEN MEAL PLANS—PALEO STYLE

I've heard people say that they thought Paleo was hard because of all the cooking. For the life of me, I cannot figure out how to get around any kind of nutritious eating without it (the cooking, that is!).

When I started seeing those dinner-assembly franchises (Dream Dinners and Super Suppers, for example) popping up all over suburbia in strip malls, and I started losing Saving Dinner subscribers, like a good student, I did my homework.

In case you're not familiar with those dinner-assembly spots, they are essentially operations that prep raw ingredients so that busy folks can assemble their meals for the week and go along their merry way.

The concept was great, but the execution? Not so much, unless you wanted a ton of carbs, bouillon, and other chemical additives in your food. Plus, those places are expensive. All you get is second-rate food that won't build your health in any way.

So, I came up with my own way to help you eat Paleo when it seems like you just don't have the time or energy to do so, by creating freezer meals.

The idea behind these freezer meals is simple: If you make them up and know they're on hand, you're less likely to fall into the "convenient" habit of doing something you'll regret later. One of my favorite ways to prepare homemade meals is by doing all the prep work ahead of time and then freezing the food raw. Then, when I decide it's time for a quick meal, all I do is thaw it, cook it, and eat it. It tastes fresh because it's not one of those icky reheated Stouffer's-type entrees from the grocery store.

Here's a little taste on the concept. With four mini-sessions to get your freezer stocked, your family will be fed in record time and you'll stay completely on plan, even when you need something in a hurry.

Freezer meals can last four to six months, depending on how they are stored. You can buy sealing systems that suck all the air out of the freezer bag, really extending the life of frozen foods. But if you follow my guidelines (which do not assume a sealing system) and use freezer-quality ziplock bags, these meals should be good in your freezer for up to four months.

All recipes have a list of assembly instructions and a corresponding recipe. I walk you through each dish, every step of the way, so all you need to do is shop for your ingredients, put the groceries away, and assemble the meals. Then, the food will be waiting for you when you need it most.

These meals are organized by protein so that you can stock up on items you find on sale, and prep a whole bunch of the same types of meals all at once. Got it? Good! Let's get started.

SEAFOOD FREEZER MEALS

Items marked with an asterisk (*) denote those needed for suggested side dishes and are, therefore, optional. Quantities will vary, depending on how often you choose to serve the suggested dish.

All of my freezer meals are accompanied by two shopping lists—one for items needed in meal assembly and one for those needed when cooking. That's because you will be doing all of the assembly at once, and you won't need the cooking ingredients until the time you choose to actually cook a particular meal.

ASSEMBLY SHOPPING LIST

PROTEIN

- Skinless salmon fillets, 6–8 oz (5)
- Skinless halibut fillets (1 lb)
- Cod fillets (1 ½ lbs)
- Shrimp (1 lb)
- Eggs (4 large)

CONDIMENTS

- Olive oil (3 tablespoons)
- Coconut oil (4 tablespoons)
- Ume plum vinegar (¼ cup)
- Raw honey (¼ cup + 1 tablespoon)

PRODUCE

- Yellow onions (2 large + 1 tablespoon minced)
- Garlic (4 cloves)
- Cauliflower (1 large)
- Carrots (1 cup grated)
- Parsley (½ cup chopped)
- Dill (¼ cup chopped)
- Lemon (2 tablespoons juice)
- Salad greens*
- Salad garnish*
- Vegetable medley to steam* (broccoli, turnips, cauliflower, etc.)
- Cauliflower*

- Kale*
- Purple potatoes*
- Vegetable medley to roast* (peppers, sweet potatoes, squash, parsnips, turnips, etc.)

SPICES

- Sea salt
- Black peppercorns
- Cayenne pepper
- Chili powder

DRY GOODS

- Blanched almond flour (1 cup)

OTHER

- Parchment paper
- Freezer bags, 1 gallon (10)

PRE-ASSEMBLY PREP LIST

PROTEIN

- Refrigerate all fish/seafood until ready to use for each recipe
- Cod fillets: Cut 1 ½ lbs into 2 oz strips
- Eggs: In a small bowl, beat 2 eggs. Set aside 2 remaining eggs (unbeaten).

CONDIMENTS

- Set out all condiments listed in Assembly Shopping List

PRODUCE

- Yellow onions: Chop and divide 2 onions, mincing 1 tablespoon
- Garlic: Mince 4 cloves in 2-clove batches
- Cauliflower: Chop 1 large head
- Carrots: Grate 1 cup
- Parsley: Chop ½ cup
- Dill: Chop ¼ cup
- Lemon: Squeeze 2 tablespoons juice

SPICES

- Set out all spices listed in Assembly Shopping List and measure as needed for each recipe

DRY GOODS

- Measure 1 cup almond flour

COOKING SHOPPING LIST

RECIPE 1: ROASTED CAULIFLOWER AND CRAB SOUP

- Chicken stock, if not using homemade (4 cups)
- Celery (2 medium stalks)
- Cooked lump crabmeat (½ lb)
- Fresh thyme (1 tablespoon chopped)
- Parchment paper

RECIPE 2: KABAYAKI SALMON

- Coconut oil (1 tablespoon)

RECIPE 3: PALEO FISH STICKS

• Ghee or coconut oil (2 tablespoons)

RECIPE 4: CUCUMBER AND SHRIMP GAZPACHO

• Cucumbers (4 large)
• Avocados (2 medium)
• Red onion (½ small)
• Olive oil (1 tablespoon)
• Lemon (2 tablespoons juice)
• Apple cider vinegar (2 tablespoons)
• Black peppercorns (¼ teaspoon freshly ground)
• Vegetable stock, if not using homemade (2 cups)
• Cilantro (2 tablespoons chopped)

RECIPE 5: PALEO GEFILTE FISH

• Ghee or coconut oil (2 tablespoons)
• Parchment paper

ASSEMBLY AND COOKING INSTRUCTIONS

Recipe 1: Roasted Cauliflower and Crab Soup

Yields 4 servings

1 large head cauliflower

2 tablespoons olive oil

1 teaspoon sea salt

1 large yellow onion, chopped

2 cloves garlic, minced

1 teaspoon freshly ground black pepper

Combine all ingredients in a 1-gallon freezer bag. Squeeze out all the air and seal the bag. To prevent freezer burn, place the filled bag in a second 1-gallon freezer bag; carefully squeeze the bag to force out any air, then seal. On the outside of the bag, label with the recipe name and date of preparation. Place it in the freezer.

BEFORE YOU COOK:

Defrost your freezer meal the night before in the fridge. If you don't have a full thaw at cooking time, remove the bag from the holding bag and place it in a sink of cold water (do not use hot water!) to speed-thaw your food safely.

COOKING INGREDIENTS:

4 cups chicken stock, preferably homemade
2 medium stalks celery, chopped
½ lb lump crabmeat, cooked
1 tablespoon chopped fresh thyme
Parchment paper

Preheat oven to 400 degrees. On a parchment-lined sheet pan, spread cauliflower mixture. Bake for 20–25 minutes or until fork-tender. Remove from oven and set aside to cool for about 10 minutes. In a food processor, pulse cauliflower mixture until it resembles grains of rice. Set aside. Place chicken stock, celery, and cauliflower mixture in a large saucepan over medium-high heat. Simmer for about 20 minutes. Add crabmeat and thyme. Cook for 5 minutes. Serve hot.

Serving suggestion: Blue Spinach Salad

Recipe 2: Kabayaki Salmon

Yields 4 servings

4 (6–8 oz) skinless salmon fillets
¼ cup ume plum vinegar
¼ cup raw honey
2 tablespoons coconut oil, melted

2 cloves garlic, minced

½ teaspoon freshly ground black pepper

Place the salmon fillets in a 1-gallon freezer bag. Set aside. In a medium bowl, whisk together remaining ingredients. Pour mixture over salmon. Squeeze out the air, seal the bag, and turn to coat. To prevent freezer burn, place the filled bag in a second 1-gallon freezer bag; carefully squeeze the bag to force out any air, then seal. On the outside of the bag, label with the recipe name and date of preparation. Place it in the freezer.

BEFORE YOU COOK:

Defrost your freezer meal the night before in the fridge. If you don't have a full thaw at cooking time, remove the bag from the holding bag and place it in a sink of cold water (do not use hot water!) to speed-thaw your food safely.

COOKING INGREDIENTS:

1 tablespoon coconut oil

COOKING INSTRUCTIONS:

Melt the coconut oil in a large skillet over medium-high heat. Remove salmon from marinade (reserving marinade) and place in the skillet. Cook for 2 minutes per side or until fillets reach desired level of doneness. Transfer salmon to a serving platter and set aside.

Pour marinade from freezer bag into a medium saucepan over medium-low heat. Cook for 4–5 minutes or until sauce bubbles and has slightly reduced. Drizzle over the cooked salmon and serve.

Serving suggestion: Cauliflower "Rice" and steamed vegetables

---

Recipe 3: Paleo Fish Sticks

Yields 4 servings

1 ½ lbs cod fillets, cut into 2 oz finger-width strips

2 large eggs, beaten

1 cup blanched almond flour

1 teaspoon sea salt

½ teaspoon freshly ground black pepper

1 pinch cayenne pepper

On a clean work surface lined with paper towels, lay out cod strips; pat dry on both sides and set aside. In a medium bowl, beat eggs and set aside. In another medium bowl, blend together remaining ingredients.

Dip each cod strip (one at a time) first in egg (shaking off any excess) and then in almond flour mixture. Place coated fish strips in a 1-gallon freezer bag, inserting parchment paper between each coated cod strip. Squeeze out air, then seal the bag. To prevent freezer burn, place the filled bag in a second 1-gallon freezer bag; carefully squeeze the bag to force out any air, then seal. On the outside of the bag, label with the recipe name and date of preparation. Place it in the freezer.

BEFORE YOU COOK:

Defrost your freezer meal the night before in the fridge. If you don't have a full thaw at cooking time, remove the bag from the holding bag and place it in a sink of cold water (do not use hot water!) to speed-thaw your food safely.

COOKING INGREDIENTS:

2 tablespoons ghee

COOKING INSTRUCTIONS:

Melt the ghee in a large skillet over medium-high heat. Add the coated cod strips and cook for 2–3 minutes per side or until golden brown on the outside and flaky on the inside. Transfer to a sheet pan lined with paper towels. Serve warm.

Serving suggestion: Mashed potatoes made with organic purple potatoes and kale salad

Recipe 4: Cucumber and Shrimp Gazpacho

Yields 4 servings

  1 lb shrimp, peeled and deveined
  1 tablespoon minced yellow onion
  1 tablespoon olive oil
  1 tablespoon fresh lemon juice
  ¼ teaspoon sea salt
  ¼ teaspoon chili powder

Place shrimp in a 1-gallon freezer bag; set aside. In a medium bowl, whisk together remaining ingredients; pour mixture over shrimp. Squeeze out all the air and seal the bag. To prevent freezer burn, place the filled bag in a second 1-gallon freezer bag; carefully squeeze the bag to force out any air, then seal. On the outside of the bag, label with the recipe name and date of preparation. Place it in the freezer.

BEFORE YOU COOK:

Defrost your freezer meal the night before in the fridge. If you don't have a full thaw at cooking time, remove the bag from the holding bag and place in a sink of cold water (do not use hot water!) to speed-thaw your food safely.

COOKING INGREDIENTS:

  4 large cucumbers, peeled, seeded, and chopped (divided)
  2 medium avocados, diced
  ½ small red onion, chopped
  1 tablespoon olive oil
  2 tablespoons fresh lemon juice
  2 tablespoons apple cider vinegar
  ½ teaspoon sea salt
  ¼ teaspoon freshly ground black pepper
  2 cups vegetable stock, preferably homemade
  2 tablespoons chopped cilantro

COOKING INSTRUCTIONS:

Preheat oven to 400 degrees. Place shrimp and marinade on a parchment-lined sheet pan; roast for 6–8 minutes or until pink and opaque. Remove from oven and set aside to cool.

In a food processor, place 3 ½ chopped cucumbers along with next 8 ingredients; puree until almost completely smooth. Pour this mixture into a large serving bowl with a lid. Chop cooled roasted shrimp and add to gazpacho mixture. Stir in remaining chopped cucumber and the cilantro. Cover and chill or serve at room temperature.

Serving suggestion: Spinach salad

Recipe 5: Paleo Gefilte Fish

Yields 4 servings

1 lb skinless halibut fillets
1 (6–8 oz) skinless salmon fillet
2 tablespoons coconut oil, melted
1 large yellow onion, chopped
2 large eggs
1 teaspoon sea salt
1 teaspoon freshly ground black pepper
1 tablespoon raw honey
1 tablespoon fresh lemon juice
¼ cup chopped fresh dill
1 cup grated carrots
½ cup chopped fresh parsley

In a food processor, pulse together first 5 ingredients until almost smooth. Add remaining ingredients and pulse until just combined. Dump this mixture into a 1-gallon freezer bag. Squeeze out the air and seal. To prevent freezer burn, place the filled bag in a second 1-gallon freezer bag; carefully squeeze the bag to force out any air, then seal. On the outside of the bag, label with the recipe name and date of preparation. Place it in the freezer.

BEFORE YOU COOK:

Defrost your freezer meal the night before in the fridge. If you don't have a full thaw at cooking time, remove the bag from the holding bag and place it in a sink of cold water (do not use hot water!) to speed-thaw your food safely.

COOKING INGREDIENTS:

2 tablespoons ghee, melted
Parchment paper

COOKING INSTRUCTIONS:

Preheat oven to 375 degrees. Line a sheet pan with parchment paper. Scoop out thawed fish mixture into 1 ½–inch balls and place on the sheet pan; brush each ball with the melted ghee and bake for 15–20 minutes or until cooked through. Serve warm.

Serving suggestion: Mashed Faux-Tatoes and roasted parsnips and red pearl onions

POULTRY FREEZER MEALS

Items marked with an asterisk (*) denote those needed for suggested side dishes and are, therefore, optional. Quantities will vary, depending on how often you choose to serve the suggested dish.

All of my freezer meals are accompanied by two shopping lists—one for items needed in meal assembly and one for those needed when cooking. That's because you will be doing all of the assembly at once, and you won't need the cooking ingredients until the time you choose to actually cook a particular meal.

ASSEMBLY SHOPPING LIST

PROTEIN

- Whole chicken (2–3 lbs)
- Boneless, skinless chicken breast halves (12)
- Boneless, skinless chicken thighs (6–8)
- Eggs (2)

CONDIMENTS

- Olive oil (2 tablespoons)
- Coconut oil (¼ cup, if not using ghee)
- Balsamic vinegar (¼ cup)
- Dijon mustard (½ cup)

PRODUCE

- Garlic (1 clove)
- Summer squash (1 cup pureed)
- Jalapeño (1 small)
- Ginger (1 tablespoon minced)
- Cilantro (1 cup chopped)
- Rosemary (4 sprigs)
- Limes (8–10 limes for 1 cup juice)
- Green apples (4)
- Salad greens*
- Salad garnish*
- Cauliflower*
- Kale*
- Sweet potatoes*
- Broccoli*

- Vegetable medley to roast* (peppers, sweet potatoes, squash, parsnips, turnips, etc.)
- Vegetable medley to stir-fry* (peppers, cabbage, beans, bok choy, carrots, etc.)

CANNED GOODS

- Diced tomatoes (14.5-oz can)
- Tomato paste (2 tablespoons)
- Unsweetened canned coconut milk (1 cup)

SPICES

- Sea salt
- Black peppercorns
- Chili powder
- Crushed red pepper flakes

DRY GOODS

- Coconut flour (½ cup)
- Unsweetened shredded coconut (¾ cup)

DAIRY

- Ghee (¼ cup, or use coconut oil)
- Parmesan cheese*

OTHER

- Parchment paper
- Freezer bags, 1 gallon (10)

PRE-ASSEMBLY PREP LIST

PROTEIN

- Refrigerate all chicken until ready to use for each recipe
- Cut up 1 (2–3 lb) whole chicken
- Cube 3 boneless, skinless chicken breast halves
- Cut 5 boneless, skinless chicken breast halves into 1-inch strips
- In a small bowl, beat 2 eggs

CONDIMENTS

- Set out all condiments as shown on Assembly Shopping List

PRODUCE

- Garlic: Mince 1 clove
- Summer squash: Roast and puree 1 cup
- Jalapeño: Seed and chop
- Ginger: Mince 1 tablespoon
- Cilantro: Chop 1 cup
- Limes: Squeeze 1 cup of juice
- Green apples: Slice

CANNED GOODS

- Open all canned goods
- Measure 2 tablespoons tomato paste
- Measure 1 cup unsweetened, canned coconut milk

SPICES

- Set out all spices as described on Assembly Shopping List and measure as needed for each recipe

DRY GOODS

- Measure ½ cup coconut flour
- Measure ¾ cup unsweetened shredded coconut

DAIRY

- Measure ¼ cup ghee (if not using coconut oil)

COOKING SHOPPING LIST

RECIPE 6: PALEO LIME AND MUSTARD CHICKEN

- Coconut oil (2 tablespoons)

RECIPE 7: STICKY COCONUTTY CHICKEN

- Rice vinegar (¾ cup)
- Raw honey (½ cup)
- Coconut aminos (3 tablespoons, see Resources)
- Crushed red pepper flakes (1 teaspoon)

RECIPE 8: ROASTED SUMMER SQUASH CHICKEN CHILI

- Chicken stock, if not using homemade (1 cup)
- Coconut oil (1 tablespoon)
- Yellow bell pepper (1 medium)

- Yellow onion (1 medium)
- Cilantro (2 tablespoons chopped)

RECIPE 9: PALEO ROSEMARY AND APPLE ROAST CHICKEN

- None

RECIPE 10: PALEO CHICKEN FINGERS

- Ghee or coconut oil (2 tablespoons)

ASSEMBLY AND COOKING INSTRUCTIONS

Recipe 6: Paleo Lime and Mustard Chicken

Yields 4 servings

4 medium boneless, skinless chicken breast halves
1 cup fresh lime juice
1 cup chopped fresh cilantro
½ cup Dijon mustard
2 tablespoons olive oil
1 tablespoon chili powder
1 teaspoon sea salt
1 teaspoon freshly ground black pepper

Place chicken in a 1-gallon freezer bag. In a food processor, pulse together remaining ingredients until almost smooth; pour mixture over chicken, squeeze out all the air in the bag, and seal. Massage the marinade into the chicken to make sure it is well coated. To prevent freezer burn, place the filled bag in a second 1-gallon freezer bag; carefully squeeze the bag to force out any air, then seal. On the outside of the bag, label with the recipe name and date of preparation. Place it in the freezer.

BEFORE YOU COOK:

Defrost your freezer meal the night before in the fridge. If you don't have a full thaw at cooking time, remove the bag from the holding bag and place it in a sink of cold water (do not use hot water!) to speed-thaw your food safely.

COOKING INGREDIENTS:

2 tablespoons coconut oil

Preheat grill to medium-high. Brush the grill grate with the coconut oil. Grill chicken for 5–7 minutes per side or until cooked through. Remove from grill and let rest at least 5 minutes before slicing and serving.

Serving suggestion: Cauliflower "Rice" and stir-fried green beans

---

Recipe 7: Sticky Coconutty Chicken

Yields 4 servings

6–8 boneless, skinless chicken thighs
1 cup canned, unsweetened coconut milk
1 tablespoon minced fresh ginger
1 teaspoon freshly ground black pepper
1 teaspoon crushed red pepper flakes

Place chicken in a 1-gallon freezer bag; pour remaining ingredients inside. Squeeze out all the air, then seal the bag. Massage the marinade into the chicken to make sure it is well coated. To prevent freezer burn, place the filled bag in a second 1-gallon freezer bag; carefully squeeze the bag to force out any air, then seal. On the outside of the bag, label with the recipe name and date of preparation. Place it in the freezer.

BEFORE YOU COOK:

Defrost your freezer meal the night before in the fridge. If you don't have a full thaw at cooking time, remove the bag from the holding bag and place it in a sink of cold water (do not use hot water!) to speed-thaw your food safely.

COOKING INGREDIENTS:

¾ cup rice vinegar

½ cup raw honey

3 tablespoons coconut aminos

1 teaspoon crushed red pepper flakes

COOKING INSTRUCTIONS:

Preheat oven to 375 degrees. Place the marinated chicken on a parchment-lined sheet pan and bake for 10–12 minutes per side.

Meanwhile, in a medium saucepan, whisk together vinegar, honey, coconut aminos, and crushed red pepper flakes. Cook over medium-high heat for 8–10 minutes or until mixture has reduced and thickened. Brush this glaze over the chicken during the last 5 minutes of baking. Remove chicken from the oven and brush with remaining glaze before serving.

Serving suggestion: Braised kale and roasted sweet potato

Recipe 8: Roasted Summer Squash Chicken Chili

Yields 4 servings

3 boneless, skinless chicken breast halves, cubed

1 cup pureed roasted summer squash

1 small jalapeño, seeded and chopped

1 (14.5 oz) can diced tomatoes with juice

2 tablespoons tomato paste

1 clove garlic, minced

1 tablespoon chili powder

1 teaspoon sea salt

Place all ingredients in a 1-gallon freezer bag. Squeeze out all the air, then seal the bag. Gently massage the bag to blend ingredients. To prevent freezer burn, place the filled bag in a second 1-gallon freezer bag; carefully squeeze the bag to force out any air, then seal. On the outside of the bag, label with the recipe name and date of preparation. Place it in the freezer.

BEFORE YOU COOK:

Defrost your freezer meal the night before in the fridge. If you don't have a full thaw at cooking time, remove the bag from the holding bag and place it in a sink of cold water (do not use hot water!) to speed-thaw your food safely.

COOKING INGREDIENTS:

1 cup chicken stock, preferably homemade

1 tablespoon coconut oil

1 medium yellow bell pepper, chopped

1 medium yellow onion, chopped

2 tablespoons chopped cilantro

COOKING INSTRUCTIONS:

Place freezer-bag ingredients in a large saucepan over medium-high heat. Stir in chicken stock. Bring to a boil, then reduce heat and allow the chili to simmer. Meanwhile, melt the coconut oil in a medium skillet over medium-high heat; add bell pepper and onion and cook until tender-crisp. Add this mixture to the chili and continue to simmer for 30–35 minutes or until chicken is cooked through. Serve with a sprinkle of chopped cilantro.

Serving suggestion: Spinach salad

Recipe 9: Paleo Rosemary and Apple Roast Chicken

Yields 4 servings

1 (2–3 lb) whole chicken, cut up

¼ cup ghee or coconut oil, melted

¼ cup balsamic vinegar

1 tablespoon sea salt

1 ½ teaspoons freshly ground black pepper

4 green apples, sliced

4 sprigs fresh rosemary

Place chicken in a 1-gallon freezer bag. In a medium bowl whisk together melted ghee or coconut oil, vinegar, salt, and pepper. Pour mixture over the chicken. Add apple slices and rosemary. Squeeze out all the air, then seal the bag. To prevent freezer burn, place the filled bag in a second 1-gallon freezer bag; carefully squeeze the bag to force out any air, then seal. On the outside of the bag, label with the recipe name and date of preparation. Place it in the freezer.

BEFORE YOU COOK:

Defrost your freezer meal the night before in the fridge. If you don't have a full thaw at cooking time, remove the bag from the holding bag and place it in a sink of cold water (do not use hot water!) to speed-thaw your food safely.

COOKING INGREDIENTS:

None

COOKING INSTRUCTIONS:

Preheat oven to 350 degrees. Place chicken and apples on a parchment-lined sheet pan. Place the rosemary sprigs under the chicken and apples. Bake for 1 hour or until chicken skin is golden and the pieces are cooked through (remember that the smaller chicken pieces cook faster and may have to be removed before the others are cooked).

Serving suggestion: Mashed Faux-Tatoes and roasted carrots, red onion, and thyme

Recipe 10: Paleo Chicken Fingers

Serves 4

2 eggs
½ cup coconut flour
½ teaspoon sea salt
¼ teaspoon freshly ground black pepper
¾ cup unsweetened shredded coconut
5 boneless, skinless chicken breast halves, cut into 1-inch strips

Beat eggs in a medium bowl. In a second medium bowl, mix coconut flour, salt, and pepper. In a third medium bowl, place the shredded coconut.

Take one chicken strip at a time and first dip into eggs, then into flour mixture. Dip the coated chicken strip once more into the egg mixture, then finally in the shredded coconut. Place the coated chicken strips in a 1-gallon freezer bag, being sure to insert a sheet of parchment paper between each strip to prevent them from sticking together. Squeeze out all the air, then seal the bag. To prevent freezer burn, place the filled bag in a second 1-gallon freezer bag; carefully squeeze the bag to force out any air, then seal. On the outside of the bag, label with the recipe name and date of preparation. Place it in the freezer.

BEFORE YOU COOK:

Defrost your freezer meal the night before in the fridge. If you don't have a full thaw at cooking time, remove the bag from the holding bag and place it in a sink of cold water (do not use hot water!) to speed-thaw your food safely.

COOKING INGREDIENTS:

2 tablespoons ghee or coconut oil, melted

COOKING INSTRUCTIONS:

Preheat oven to 400 degrees. Place coated chicken strips on a parchment-lined sheet pan, leaving a little space between each. Drizzle the melted ghee or coconut oil on top. Bake for 15–25 minutes or until chicken strips are golden brown on the outside and cooked through on the inside. Serve warm.

Serving suggestion: Spinach salad and steamed broccoli

BEEF FREEZER MEALS

Items marked with an asterisk (*) denote those needed for suggested side dishes and are, therefore, optional. Quantities will vary, depending on how often you choose to serve the suggested dish.

All of my freezer meals are accompanied by two shopping lists—one for items needed in meal assembly and one for those needed when cooking. That's because you will be doing all of the assembly at once, and you won't need the cooking ingredients until the time you choose to actually cook a particular meal.

ASSEMBLY SHOPPING LIST

PROTEIN

- Beef inside skirt steak (2 lbs)
- Beef flank steak (2 lbs)
- Ground beef (3 lbs)

CONDIMENTS

- Coconut oil (2 tablespoons)
- Coconut cream (½ cup)
- Ghee (½ cup)
- Coconut aminos (¾ cup + 2 tablespoons, see Resources)
- Thai fish sauce (1 tablespoon, in Asian section of grocery store)
- Hot chili sauce (1 teaspoon, in Asian section of grocery store)
- Sun-dried tomatoes, packed in olive oil (¾ cup chopped)
- Raw honey (½ cup)

PRODUCE

- Yellow onions (2 medium)
- Garlic (10 cloves plus 2 tablespoons minced)
- Ginger (3 teaspoons grated)
- Basil (2 cups + 2 tablespoons chopped)
- Thai basil (1 bunch)
- Chives (2 tablespoons chopped)
- Lime (1 medium)
- Sweet potatoes*

- Salad greens*
- Salad garnish*
- Potatoes*
- Brussels sprouts*

CANNED GOODS

- Beef broth, if not using homemade (1 cup)
- Diced tomatoes (2 14.5-oz cans)
- Tomato paste (2 tablespoons)

SPICES

- Sea salt
- Black peppercorns
- Cayenne pepper
- Crushed red pepper flakes

DRY GOODS

- Arrowroot powder (½ cup)
- Walnut halves (1 cup)

OTHER

- Freezer bags (10 1-gallon bags and 1 1-quart bag)

PRE-ASSEMBLY PREP LIST

PROTEIN

- Keep all meat refrigerated until ready to use for each recipe
- Cut 2 lbs beef flank steak into strips

CONDIMENTS

• Set out all condiments as described in Assembly Shopping List and measure as needed for each recipe

PRODUCE

• Yellow onions: Chop 2
• Garlic: Mince as needed for each recipe
• Ginger: Grate 3 teaspoons
• Basil: Chop 2 tablespoons
• Thai basil: Chop 1 bunch
• Chives: Chop 2 tablespoons
• Lime: Squeeze juice from 1

CANNED GOODS

• Measure 1 cup beef broth
• Open 2 cans diced tomatoes
• Measure 2 tablespoons tomato paste

SPICES

• Set out all spices as described on Assembly Shopping List and measure as needed for each recipe

DRY GOODS

• Measure ½ cup arrowroot powder

COOKING SHOPPING LIST

RECIPE 11: BEEF THAI BASIL LETTUCE WRAPS

- Coconut oil (2 tablespoons)
- Red bell pepper (1 large)
- Thai basil (2 tablespoons chopped)
- Butter lettuce (12 medium leaves)

RECIPE 12: SUN-DRIED TOMATO MEATBALLS WITH PESTO

- Coconut oil (2 tablespoons)
- Parchment paper

RECIPE 13: GINGER BEEF AND MANGO SALSA

- Coconut oil (2 tablespoons)
- Green mango (1 cup chopped)
- Red onion (½ small)
- Avocado (1)
- Cilantro (⅓ cup chopped)
- Ginger (½ teaspoon grated)
- Garlic powder (1 teaspoon)
- Lime (1 tablespoon juice)

RECIPE 14: SPAGHETTI SQUASH WITH BEEF BOLOGNESE SAUCE

- Coconut oil (1 tablespoon)
- Ground beef (1 lb)
- Sea salt (1 teaspoon)
- Black peppercorns (½ teaspoon freshly ground)

- Spaghetti squash (1 large)
- Fresh basil (2 tablespoons chopped)

RECIPE 15: MONGOLIAN BEEF

- Coconut oil (½ cup)
- Green onions (3)

ASSEMBLY AND COOKING INSTRUCTIONS

Recipe 11: Beef Thai Basil Lettuce Wraps

Yields 4 servings

    1 ½ lbs ground beef
    1 medium yellow onion, chopped
    1 bunch Thai basil, chopped
    2 cloves garlic, minced
    2 tablespoons coconut aminos
    1 teaspoon hot chili sauce
    1 medium lime, juiced

In a large bowl, combine ground beef, onion, and basil; set aside. In a small bowl, whisk together remaining ingredients; pour over beef mixture and gently blend together. Place this mixture into a 1-gallon freezer bag. Squeeze out all the air, then seal the bag. To prevent freezer burn, place the filled bag in a second 1-gallon freezer bag; carefully squeeze the bag to force out any air, then seal. On the outside of the bag, label with the recipe name and date of preparation. Place it in the freezer.

BEFORE YOU COOK:

Defrost your freezer meal the night before in the fridge. If you don't have a full thaw at cooking time, remove the bag from the holding bag and place it in a sink of cold water (do not use hot water!) to speed-thaw your food safely.

COOKING INGREDIENTS:

2 tablespoons coconut oil

1 large red bell pepper, chopped

2 tablespoons chopped Thai basil

12 medium butter lettuce leaves

COOKING INSTRUCTIONS:

Melt coconut oil in a large skillet over medium-high heat. Add beef mixture and cook, breaking up meat with a wooden spoon, until no longer pink. Add bell pepper and cook until tender-crisp. Remove skillet from heat and add Thai basil. Scoop cooked beef mixture into lettuce leaves and serve.

Serving suggestion: Roasted sweet potato

Recipe 12: Sun-dried Tomato Meatballs with Pesto

Yields 4 servings

MEATBALLS:

1 ½ lbs ground beef

2 tablespoons chopped fresh chives

2 tablespoons chopped fresh basil

½ cup chopped sun-dried tomatoes, packed in olive oil

2 cloves garlic, minced

1 teaspoon sea salt

1 teaspoon freshly ground black pepper

PESTO:

1 cup walnut halves

½ cup ghee, melted

2 cloves garlic, minced

½ teaspoon sea salt

2 cups fresh basil

¼ cup sun-dried tomatoes

½ cup coconut cream

In a large bowl, mix together all ingredients for meatballs; form mixture into 1 ½–inch balls. Place meatballs in layers in a 1-gallon freezer bag, inserting a piece of parchment paper between each layer. Squeeze out all the air, then seal the bag. To prevent freezer burn, place the filled bag in a second 1-gallon freezer bag; carefully squeeze the bag to force out any air, then seal. On the outside of the bag, label with the recipe name and date of preparation.

To prepare pesto: Place all ingredients in a food processor and process until smooth. Place in a separate zipper-style plastic bag. Squeeze out all the air, then seal the bag. Place the pesto bag inside the holding bag with the meatballs. Place in freezer.

BEFORE YOU COOK:

Defrost your freezer meal the night before in the fridge. If you don't have a full thaw at cooking time, remove the bag from the holding bag and place it in a sink of cold water (do not use hot water!) to speed-thaw your food safely.

COOKING INGREDIENTS:

2 tablespoons coconut oil, melted

Parchment paper

COOKING INSTRUCTIONS:

Preheat oven to 375 degrees. Place meatballs on a parchment-lined sheet pan so that none are touching, and drizzle melted coconut oil over the top. Bake for 15–20 minutes or until browned on the outside and cooked through on the inside. Remove from oven and keep warm. Drizzle pesto over meatballs and serve.

Serving suggestion: Spaghetti squash and a spinach salad

Recipe 13: Ginger Beef and Mango Salsa

Yields 4 servings

   2 lbs beef inside skirt steaks
   ¼ cup coconut aminos
   1 tablespoon Thai fish sauce
   1 teaspoon grated ginger
   ¼ teaspoon cayenne pepper
   ½ teaspoon freshly ground black pepper

Place steaks in a 1-gallon freezer bag; set aside. In a medium bowl, whisk together remaining ingredients; pour mixture over steaks. Squeeze out all the air, then seal the bag and gently massage it to work the marinade into the meat. To prevent freezer burn, place the filled bag in a second 1-gallon freezer bag; carefully squeeze the bag to force out any air, then seal. On the outside of the bag, label with the recipe name and date of preparation. Place it in the freezer.

BEFORE YOU COOK:

Defrost your freezer meal the night before in the fridge. If you don't have a full thaw at cooking time, remove the bag from the holding bag and place it in a sink of cold water (do not use hot water!) to speed-thaw your food safely.

COOKING INGREDIENTS:

   2 tablespoons coconut oil, melted
   1 cup chopped green mango
   ½ small red onion, thinly sliced
   1 avocado, diced
   ⅓ cup chopped cilantro
   ½ teaspoon grated ginger
   1 teaspoon garlic powder
   1 tablespoon freshly squeezed lime juice

COOKING INSTRUCTIONS:

Preheat grill to medium-high. Brush grill grate with melted coconut oil. Place marinated steaks on the grill and cook for 2–4 minutes per side or until they reach desired level of doneness. Remove steaks from the grill and let them rest for at least 10 minutes.

To prepare salsa: In a medium bowl, combine remaining ingredients; serve over steaks.

Serving suggestion: Sautéed yellow squash and zucchini

Recipe 14: Spaghetti Squash with Beef Bolognese Sauce

Yields 4 servings

- 2 tablespoons tomato paste
- 1 (14.5 oz) can diced tomatoes
- 4 cloves garlic, minced
- 1 medium yellow onion, chopped
- 2 teaspoons sea salt
- 1 teaspoon freshly ground black pepper

In a large bowl, combine all ingredients; pour mixture into a 1-gallon freezer bag. Squeeze out all the air, then seal the bag. To prevent freezer burn, place the filled bag in a second 1-gallon freezer bag; carefully squeeze the bag to force out any air, then seal. On the outside of the bag, label with the recipe name and date of preparation. Place it in the freezer.

BEFORE YOU COOK:

Defrost your freezer meal the night before in the fridge. If you don't have a full thaw at cooking time, remove the bag from the holding bag and place it in a sink of cold water (do not use hot water!) to speed-thaw your food safely.

COOKING INGREDIENTS:

1 tablespoon coconut oil

1 lb ground beef

1 teaspoon sea salt

½ teaspoon freshly ground black pepper

1 large spaghetti squash, roasted, seeded, and "noodles" scraped out

2 tablespoons chopped fresh basil

COOKING INSTRUCTIONS:

Place contents of freezer bag in a large saucepan over medium-high heat; bring to a boil, then reduce heat and simmer. Meanwhile, melt coconut oil in a medium skillet over medium-high heat. Add ground beef. Cook, breaking up meat with a wooden spoon, until no longer pink. Season with salt and pepper, then add to tomato mixture; continue to simmer for 20 minutes. Serve sauce over spaghetti squash "noodles" and top with chopped basil.

Serving suggestion: Spinach salad

Recipe 15: Mongolian Beef

Yields 4 servings

½ cup arrowroot powder

1 teaspoon sea salt, divided

1 teaspoon freshly ground black pepper, divided

2 lbs beef flank steak, cut into strips

2 tablespoons coconut oil, melted

2 tablespoons minced garlic

2 teaspoons grated fresh ginger

1 pinch crushed red pepper flakes

½ cup coconut aminos

1 cup beef broth, preferably homemade

½ cup raw honey, melted

In a medium bowl, blend together arrowroot powder, ½ teaspoon salt, and ½ teaspoon pepper; dredge steak strips in this mixture, shaking off any excess. Place coated steak strips in a 1-gallon freezer bag. Squeeze out all the air and seal the bag. In a medium bowl, whisk together the remaining ingredients, along with remaining salt and pepper. Pour mixture into a 1-quart freezer bag. Squeeze out all the air and seal the bag. To prevent freezer burn, place the filled bags in a second 1-gallon freezer bag; carefully squeeze the bag to force out any air, then seal. On the outside of the bag, label with the recipe name and date of preparation. Place it in the freezer.

BEFORE YOU COOK:

Defrost your freezer meal the night before in the fridge. If you don't have a full thaw at cooking time, remove the bags from the holding bag and place them in a sink of cold water (do not use hot water!) to speed-thaw your food safely.

COOKING INGREDIENTS:

½ cup coconut oil
3 green onions, chopped

COOKING INSTRUCTIONS:

Place the contents of the 1-quart freezer bag in a medium saucepan over medium-low heat. Bring to a low bowl, then simmer for 10–15 minutes or until slightly reduced and thickened; set aside.

Melt the coconut oil in a large skillet over medium-high heat. Add steak strips and cook for 2–3 minutes per side or until they reach desired level of doneness. Pour the cooked sauce over the steak strips and garnish with chopped green onions.

Serving suggestion: A big mixed-greens salad with your favorite fixings

PORK FREEZER MEALS

Items marked with an asterisk (*) denote those needed for suggested side dishes and are, therefore, optional. Quantities will vary, depending on how often you choose to serve the suggested dish.

All of my freezer meals are accompanied by two shopping lists—one for items needed in meal assembly and one for those needed when cooking. That's because you will be doing all of the assembly at once, and you won't need the cooking ingredients until the time you choose to actually cook a particular meal.

ASSEMBLY SHOPPING LIST

PROTEIN

- Bacon (5 slices)
- Pork tenderloin (1 ½ lbs)
- Boneless top loin pork chops (4 6-oz chops or 1 ½ lbs)
- Boneless pork shoulder (1 ½ lbs)
- Smoked ham hock (1 medium)
- Ground pork (1 lb)
- Egg (1)

CONDIMENTS

- Ghee (4–5 tablespoons)
- Coconut oil (1 tablespoon)
- Thai fish sauce (2 ½ tablespoons)
- Coconut aminos (½ tablespoon, see Resources)

PRODUCE

- Mushrooms (½ cup sliced)
- Portobello mushrooms (2 large)
- Yellow onions (5)
- Garlic (5–6 cloves)
- Red bell peppers (3)
- Red chili (1 tablespoon chopped)

- Spinach (2 cups chopped)
- Carrots (1 cup shredded)
- Celery (¼ cup chopped)
- Lettuce leaves (16 small)
- Lemon (1)
- Green apple (1 medium)
- Green beans*
- Cauliflower*
- Broccoli*
- Purple potatoes*
- Spinach*
- Sweet potatoes*

CANNED GOODS

- Low-sodium beef broth (2 ½ cups)
- Low-sodium chicken broth (½ cup)
- Unsweetened coconut milk (3 tablespoons + 1 ½ cups)

SPICES

- Sea salt
- Freshly ground black pepper
- Bay leaves (2)
- Fresh rosemary (1 tablespoon chopped)
- Fresh thyme (1 tablespoon chopped)
- Fresh parsley (1 tablespoon)
- Fresh cilantro (1 ¼ cups chopped)
- Fresh ginger (3 tablespoons grated)
- Ground cumin
- Arrowroot powder
- Curry powder
- Ground cinnamon

DRY GOODS

- Dried shiitake mushrooms (3)
- Coconut flour (2 tablespoons)

FREEZER

- Chopped spinach (1 cup)

OTHER

- Kitchen string
- Parchment paper

PRE-ASSEMBLY PREP LIST

PROTEIN

- Keep all meat refrigerated until ready to use for each recipe
- Chop 2 slices of bacon
- On a clean work surface, butterfly pork tenderloin so the meat lies flat like a book; cover in plastic wrap and pound flat
- Cut 4 top sirloin pork chops into strips
- Cut pork shoulder into 1-inch cubes
- Cut 4 pork chops into 1-inch pieces

CONDIMENTS

- Set out all condiments as described in Assembly Shopping List and measure as needed for each recipe

PRODUCE

- Mushrooms: Slice ½ cup
- Dried shiitake mushrooms: Reconstitute and chop 3
- Large portobello mushrooms: Slice 2
- Red bell peppers: Slice 2 medium and 1 small
- Yellow onion: Chop 2 + ¼ cup and thinly slice 2
- Celery: Chop ¼ cup
- Cilantro: Chop ¼ cup
- Granny Smith apple: Peel, core, and chop 1
- Ginger: Grate 3 tablespoons
- Carrots: Shred 1 cup
- Red chili: Chop 1 tablespoon
- Frozen chopped spinach: Thaw and drain 1 cup
- Garlic: Mince 5 cloves
- Fresh spinach: Chop 2 cups
- Fresh rosemary: Chop 1 tablespoon
- Fresh thyme: Chop 1 tablespoon

CANNED GOODS

- Measure ½ cup chicken stock
- Measure 3 tablespoons canned coconut milk

SPICES

- Set out all spices as described on Assembly Shopping List and measure as needed for each recipe

DRY GOODS

- Measure 2 tablespoons coconut flour
- Measure 1 teaspoon arrowroot powder

COOKING SHOPPING LIST

RECIPE 16: PALEO STUFFED PORK TENDERLOIN

- Ghee (2 tablespoons)
- Lemon (zest 1 teaspoon)
- Fresh parsley (1 tablespoon, chopped)
- Sea salt (¼ teaspoon)
- Freshly ground pepper (1 pinch)

RECIPE 17: SPICY THAI PORK STIR-FRY

- Ghee (2 tablespoons)

RECIPE 18: BRAZILIAN PORK STEW

- Ghee (2 tablespoons)
- Smoked ham hock (1)
- Bay leaves (2)
- Beef broth (2 ½ cups, though homemade is best)
- Fresh cilantro (½ cup, chopped)

RECIPE 19: GREEN PORK SLIDERS

- Coconut oil (2 tablespoons)
- Small lettuce leaves (16)

RECIPE 20: PORK AND APPLE CURRY

- Coconut oil (2 tablespoons)
- Unsweetened canned coconut milk (1 ½ cups)
- Cilantro (½ cup, chopped)

ASSEMBLY AND COOKING INSTRUCTIONS

Recipe 16: Paleo Stuffed Pork Tenderloin

Yields 4 servings

> 2 slices bacon, chopped
>
> ½ cup sliced mushrooms
>
> 1 yellow onion, chopped
>
> 2 cloves garlic, minced
>
> 2 cups chopped fresh spinach
>
> 1 tablespoon chopped fresh rosemary
>
> 1 tablespoon chopped fresh thyme
>
> ½ teaspoon sea salt
>
> ½ teaspoon freshly ground black pepper
>
> 1 ½ lbs pork tenderloin
>
> Kitchen string

Cook bacon in a medium skillet on medium-high heat until crisp; remove from pan and set aside, leaving drippings in the pan. Add mushrooms, onion, and garlic; cook until onion is slightly browned. Add spinach and cook just until wilted. Remove skillet from heat and add chopped bacon, rosemary, thyme, salt, and pepper; set aside.

Spread bacon/spinach mixture over flattened tenderloin, and then roll the tenderloin up so that the filling spirals inside. Secure tenderloin with kitchen string; place in a 1-gallon freezer bag. Squeeze out the air and seal the bag. To prevent freezer burn, place the filled bag in a second 1-gallon freezer bag; carefully squeeze the bag to force out any air, then seal. On the outside of the bag, label with the recipe name and date of preparation. Place it in the freezer.

BEFORE YOU COOK:

Defrost your freezer meal the night before in the fridge. If you don't have a full thaw at cooking time, remove the bag from the holding bag and place it in a sink of cold water (do not use hot water!) to speed-thaw your food safely.

COOKING INGREDIENTS:

Parchment paper

2 tablespoons ghee, melted

1 teaspoon lemon zest

1 tablespoon chopped fresh parsley

¼ teaspoon sea salt

1 pinch freshly ground black pepper

COOKING INSTRUCTIONS:

Preheat oven to 375 degrees. Place pork tenderloin on a parchment-lined sheet pan and bake for 45 minutes or until cooked through. Remove from the oven and set aside to rest for at least 10 minutes before slicing.

In a medium bowl, whisk together remaining ingredients; drizzle over sliced pork and serve.

Serving suggestion: Roasted green beans with crushed red pepper and garlic

---

Recipe 17: Spicy Thai Pork Stir-Fry

Yields 4 servings

2 medium red bell peppers, sliced

2 tablespoons Thai fish sauce

1 large yellow onion, sliced

1 ½ lbs boneless top loin pork chops, cut into strips

3 tablespoons grated fresh ginger

1 cup shredded carrots

1 tablespoon chopped red chili

Place all ingredients in a 1-gallon freezer bag. Squeeze out all the air, then seal the bag. Shake gently to mix well. To prevent freezer burn, place the filled bag in a second 1-gallon freezer bag; carefully squeeze the bag to force out any air, then seal. On the outside of the bag, label with the recipe name and date of preparation. Place it in the freezer.

BEFORE YOU COOK:

Defrost your freezer meal the night before in the fridge. If you don't have a full thaw at cooking time, remove the bag from the holding bag and place it in a sink of cold water (do not use hot water!) to speed-thaw your food safely.

COOKING INGREDIENTS:

2 tablespoons ghee

COOKING INSTRUCTIONS:

Melt the ghee in a large skillet over medium-high heat. Add contents of freezer bag; cook and stir until pork is cooked through and vegetables are tender-crisp. Remove from heat and serve.

Serving suggestion: Cauliflower "Rice" and steamed asparagus

Recipe 18: Brazilian Pork Stew

1 yellow onion, chopped
2 cloves garlic, minced
3 slices bacon, cooked and chopped
1 ½ lbs boneless pork shoulder, cut into 1-inch cubes
1 teaspoon ground cumin
2 large portobello mushrooms, sliced
2 teaspoons sea salt
1 teaspoon freshly ground black pepper

Place all ingredients in a 1-gallon freezer bag. Squeeze out all the air, then seal the bag. Shake the bag to blend ingredients well. To prevent freezer burn, place the filled bag in a second 1-gallon freezer bag; carefully squeeze the bag to force out any air, then seal. On the outside of the bag, label with the recipe name and date of preparation. Place it in the freezer.

BEFORE YOU COOK:

Defrost your freezer meal the night before in the fridge. If you don't have a full thaw at cooking time, remove the bag from the holding bag and place it in a sink of cold water (do not use hot water!) to speed-thaw your food safely.

COOKING INGREDIENTS:

2 tablespoons ghee
1 smoked ham hock
2 bay leaves
2 ½ cups beef broth, preferably homemade
½ cup chopped cilantro

COOKING INSTRUCTIONS:

Melt ghee in a large saucepan with a tight-fitting lid over medium-high heat. Add contents of freezer bag; cook and stir until pork is cooked through and vegetables are tender-crisp. Add ham hock, bay leaves, and broth. Bring mixture to a boil, then reduce heat, cover, and simmer for 1 ½–2 hours, stirring occasionally and adding more liquid if necessary. Remove ham hock and bay leaves. When ham hock is cool enough to handle, chop the meat off the bone and add to soup. Serve soup sprinkled with chopped cilantro.

Serving suggestion: Sautéed broccoli and cauliflower with cumin and red pepper flakes

---

Recipe 19: Green Pork Sliders

Yields 4 servings

1 cup frozen chopped spinach, thawed and drained
1 tablespoon coconut oil
¼ cup chopped yellow onion
3 dried shiitake mushrooms, reconstituted and chopped
3 tablespoons unsweetened coconut milk
¼ cup chopped celery

¼ cup chopped fresh cilantro

1 lb ground pork

1 egg, beaten

2 tablespoons coconut flour

½ tablespoon Thai fish sauce

½ tablespoon coconut aminos

½ teaspoon sea salt

1 teaspoon freshly ground black pepper

In a large bowl, combine all ingredients; form mixture into 8 small patties. Place the patties in a single layer in a 1-gallon freezer bag, inserting parchment paper between layers. Squeeze out all the air, then seal the bag. To prevent freezer burn, place the filled bag in a second 1-gallon freezer bag; carefully squeeze the bag to force out any air, then seal. On the outside of the bag, label with the recipe name and date of preparation. Place it in the freezer.

BEFORE YOU COOK:

Defrost your freezer meal the night before in the fridge. If you don't have a full thaw at cooking time, remove the bag from the holding bag and place it in a sink of cold water (do not use hot water!) to speed-thaw your food safely.

COOKING INGREDIENTS:

2 tablespoons coconut oil

16 small lettuce leaves

COOKING INSTRUCTIONS:

Preheat grill to medium-high. Brush grill grate with coconut oil. Grill slider patties for 2–4 minutes per side or until cooked through. Remove from heat and place a patty between two lettuce leaves. Serve with your favorite burger condiments.

Serving suggestion: Leanne's Quick Garlicky Spinach (In a large skillet, heat olive oil over medium heat. Once hot, cook fresh minced garlic and a tub of fresh baby spinach until it wilts completely. Season with sea salt and freshly ground black pepper.)

Recipe 20: Pork and Apple Curry

Yields 4 servings

2 tablespoons ghee, melted

4 (6 oz) boneless pork chops, cut into 1-inch pieces

1 small yellow onion, thinly sliced

1 clove garlic, minced

1 Granny Smith apple, peeled, cored, and chopped

1 small red bell pepper, sliced

½ cup chicken stock, preferably homemade

1 teaspoon arrowroot powder

1 teaspoon curry powder

½ teaspoon ground cumin

½ teaspoon ground cinnamon

2 teaspoons sea salt

1 teaspoon freshly ground black pepper

In a large bowl, toss together all ingredients until pork is evenly coated. Place this mixture in a 1-gallon freezer bag. Squeeze out all the air, then seal the bag. To prevent freezer burn, place the filled bag in a second 1-gallon freezer bag; carefully squeeze the bag to force out any air, then seal. On the outside of the bag, label with the recipe name and date of preparation. Place it in the freezer.

BEFORE YOU COOK:

Defrost your freezer meal the night before in the fridge. If you don't have a full thaw at cooking time, remove the bag from the holding bag and place it in a sink of cold water (do not use hot water!) to speed-thaw your food safely.

COOKING INGREDIENTS:

2 tablespoons coconut oil

1 ½ cups unsweetened coconut milk

½ cup cilantro, chopped

COOKING INSTRUCTIONS:

Melt coconut oil in a large skillet over medium-high heat. Add pork mixture and cook until heated through. Add coconut milk and continue to cook until mixture comes to a simmer and thickens into a sauce. To serve, sprinkle with chopped cilantro.

And now I've added twenty dishes to your arsenal for those crazy nights when you need to count on your freezer to get dinner on the table.

10

CHAPTER TEN
THE PART-TIME PALEO FAMILY

I don't have many regrets in life, but I sure do wish I had known more about the benefits of avoiding grains, gluten, legumes, and dairy back when my kids were little. I'm a nutritionist, so we've always eaten very well—my kids love their veggies—but they were raised on plenty of whole-grain breads and a fair bit of brown rice, too.

I don't lose any sleep over this and you shouldn't either if you're in the same boat. My children are healthy and happy young adults. Regardless of the age of your child or what his or her diet currently looks like, there are many health benefits in going Paleo. A Part-Time Paleo diet often leads to fewer allergies, lower incidence of diabetes, and lower chance of obesity.

If you have any concerns about transitioning your child to a Part-Time Paleo diet, make an appointment to consult with a pediatrician. Otherwise, jump right in!

Depending on your family's starting point, this transition might be challenging. But what's the point of eating better if you continue feeding your family foods that aren't good for them? I know it's a lot easier said than done to change the way your loved ones eat—especially kids.

That's why I think the earlier you can get them onto a healthy path, the better.

When children are very young, they're just starting to form their food associations and their eating habits. If you nourish them with fresh produce, fruits, nuts, and lean meats, they will grow up knowing how good those foods make them feel. And on the other side of the equation, they'll also learn quickly how eating processed, sugar-laden foods makes them feel like crap.

The reality is the majority of American kids today are used to eating typical "kid" foods, which, really, should be referred to as "foodlike items," because as far as I'm concerned, hot dogs and neon orange mac and cheese are not food.

So, how do you go about changing those habits?

You don't do it all at once, that's for sure. Don't make a big announcement to your family. Make the Part-Time Paleo thing a nonissue. Don't put a name on it at all. At home, just start serving up your new, healthier dishes and wait to see if they notice. They probably will realize that they no longer eat toast and peanut butter for breakfast, but they might enjoy the big fruit salad and scoop of Greek yogurt with a drizzle of honey even more. If they're used to eating cold cereal for breakfast, they might enjoy a switch to bacon and eggs! Do explain why you're eating all of those extra vegetables every single day—because they give us all of the nutrients we need to grow big and tall with strong teeth and shiny hair—but don't draw attention to the items that are missing.

If there are no crackers or cookies in the kitchen, your family members can't eat them. Give those fellow grocery-store shoppers cart envy by piling your bags with produce, not packaged snacks. Then, when you get home and everyone starts asking for snacks, their only options will be foods that will nourish their bodies, not detract from their health.

MAKING THE TRANSITION TO PART-TIME PALEO

You will need to prioritize avoiding gluten-containing grains. (Did you know gluten is associated with learning disorders?) As you start to transition your family to Part-Time Paleo, find as many substitutions for family favorites as you can to help make it a bit easier. If your crew eats sandwiches three times a day, cut out one sandwich and make the others on gluten-free bread. Do that for one week, then cut out the second sandwich. See where I'm going with this? (Isn't it refreshing to have so much leeway on a "diet"?)

Dairy is avoided by most Paleoistas, but when it comes to kids, milk is a touchy subject and you should use your own judgment. Fermented dairy products, like plain Greek yogurt and cheese aged more than 120 days, are preferable over milk; if you're hesitant about giving up all dairy, those options will work. If you choose to continue to give your children milk, buy organic because of the high amounts of hormones and antibiotics found in conventional milk. And buy full-fat milk. It's better for them than the more processed 1%, 2%, and skim varieties.

The one area where all Part-Time Paleoistas and Paleo purists will agree is that vegetables are king. Get as much organic produce into your family as you possibly can. Get the kids involved in the grocery shopping, so they can select which foods they'd like to try. Tell your kids you need two green vegetables, a yellow vegetable, a purple fruit, and two orange items, and see what they come up with. Let them choose between almonds and walnuts. Besides getting them excited about the foods they'd like to try, you'll be giving them the life skill of knowing how to shop.

Once you get those ingredients home, have everyone pitch in and help out in the kitchen so they're involved in the food preparation process: hands-on nutrition! They'll eat what they make—great trick!

CREATIVE WAYS TO GET MORE VEGGIES INTO YOUR LIFE

It's easy to eat fruit. Fruit is sweet and it comes in pretty colors. Vegetables, though? Well that's a whole other story.

There are dozens of ways to increase your veggie intake. Puree vegetables into spaghetti sauce and soups. Put pumpkin puree in your beef stew. Grate beets into beef burritos. Keep veggies "omnipresent" with every meal, whether they're seen or not.

Here are a few creative ways you can get more vegetables into your family's diet.

- **Make it fun.** Serve snacks like ants on a log. Spread almond butter or sunflower butter on a piece of washed, organic celery, and place raisins (ants) walking down the log. Place an assortment of sliced veggies in different shapes on a plate and encourage your children to make art out of their food. Who can make a funny face out of their veggies? Extra points for eating your own creation!
- **Offer veggies when kids are hungry.** Sounds obvious, but kids will eat what they're offered when they're hungry. If you put out a bowl of chips, of course the kids will eat them. But if you put out a plate of veggies and celery sticks to snack on, they'll eat them, too, if that's their only option!
- **Involve them.** When you make a salad, instead of bringing it to the table in a big bowl, present your family members with veggies in separate bowls and let everyone choose which ones they want.
- **Introduce new vegetables in foods they already love.** If your kids love soup, make a big pot and add a new vegetable in there. If everyone around the dinner table goes ape for gluten-free pasta, add some broccoli to your next batch. If meatloaf is something everyone in your house loves, grate some veggies into it. Yes, this sounds like hiding veggies, but there's nothing wrong with adding nutrients to dishes your kids already love. Just be sure to tell them while they're gobbling up what's in there. That will make it more likely they'll try those veggies in other forms as well!
- **Let them drink it.** Toss some kale, carrots, and any other veggies you have on hand into the juicer. For sweetness, add an apple. Toss in some fresh ginger for an added nutritional boost. Serve with a straw in a pretty glass and voilà!

All of these strategies worked for my two kids (now in their twenties), and they'll eat any veggie that's put in front of them!

Find healthy swaps for family favorites. Instead of buying those nitrate-packed hot dog wieners, buy brands like Boar's Head or Applegate Farms. Ditch the artificially colored mac and cheese (the familiar bright orange brand we all know has been banned in the UK because it contains proven carcinogenic colorants), and find a nice organic gluten-free pasta like buckwheat or quinoa. Paleo purists would hang me up for suggesting such a thing, but you still need to transition your children. In place of that powdered cheese, drizzle the noodles with butter or olive oil and let them top it with a nice real cheese, some diced chicken, and organic green peas. By the way, peas are also non-Paleo, but they are naturally sweet, which kids like, plus they have all kinds of nutrition, including protein.

When you're going Part-Time Paleo (especially with kids), you'll need to forget what you used to think about meals. This lifestyle gives you the freedom to stray from the confines of what you used to believe about meals (back around the time you opened this book for the first time). I hear people say all the time that they can't figure out how to do Paleo for breakfast when they can't feed everyone cereal with milk.

What will they do for lunch when they can't have a sandwich?

When you follow the Part-Time Paleo way of life, you will find that your idea of meals changes. There's nothing wrong with having a fried egg with a grass-fed burger patty topped with avocado and tomato for breakfast. Food is food, and it doesn't matter what you eat when. Don't stress out over the thought of not packing a sandwich in the lunch box. Choose a variety of your kids' favorite proteins, fruits, and vegetables, and pack the box full!

We know that kids will be kids. There will be birthday parties with candy and sweets, and Grandma will still try to shove cookies at them, so it's okay to stick to a Part-Time Paleo diet at home and loosen up when it comes to those other sorts of activities.

When you eat well at home and you know that your children are getting the best food you can provide for them, it makes it easier to swallow (pun intended) when they're munching down on high-fructose corn syrup at Grandma's house. But you know what? Your kids might end up surprising you. Once they get used to this lifestyle, they might just gravitate away from the foods you no longer allow at home.

PALEO SNACKS

I detest those 100-calorie snack packs you find in grocery stores nowadays. Those packages are full of highly processed foods—heavy on sugar and chemicals. Here's a list of easy substitute snack ideas!

1. Raw veggies and dip: Experiment with cauliflower, broccoli, and pepper strips
2. Celery sticks with almond butter and raisins (ants on a log!)
3. Homemade trail mix: Mixing dried fruit and nuts couldn't be easier
4. Sliced apple and blueberries, sprinkled with cinnamon
5. Mixed berries: Strawberries, blackberries, and blueberries make a wonderful snack
6. Muffins: Bake your own Paleo muffins with fruit and flax and other good things
7. Banana: The perfect snack—with almond butter, it can be deliciously filling
8. Cheese: A few cubes of aged cheese make a wonderful snack
9. Nuts: A handful of nuts provides an excellent protein boost
10. Popsicles: Invest in some of those plastic popsicle molds and fill them with homemade juices or yogurt mixed with fruit
11. Yogurt: Buy plain Greek yogurt and sweeten it with fruit to avoid unnecessary sugar—this is Primal, not Paleo, and would qualify as a Part-Time Paleo snack
12. Cucumbers: Make a sandwich out of cucumber slices and cream cheese
13. Homemade granola bars: Find a recipe that your family will love and create your own version of this lunch box staple
14. Dried fruit: Dried apricots, dates, cranberries, and pineapple are loaded with fiber and minerals
15. Banana bread: Experiment with nut flour recipes low in sugar until you find the one your family loves best
16. Boiled eggs

17. Applesauce: Core and slice some organic apples, simmer them down, and sprinkle with cinnamon. Ta-da . . . applesauce!
18. Orange: An orange is another great snack that comes in its own biodegradable wrapper!
19. Grapes: Wash some organic grapes and snip off a bunch for a delicious sweet treat
20. Melons: Make a salad of honeydew, cantaloupe, and watermelon
21. Broccoli trees
22. Fruit kebabs: Make fruit more fun by sticking it on a skewer! Provide Greek yogurt for dipping.
23. Almond butter: Apple slices, bananas, and celery are all great friends of almond butter
24. Kale chips: How much healthier can you get than kale? Make a batch of kale chips and see how fast they disappear.
25. Sweet potato fries: Slice some sweet potatoes and bake them on a rack for a fast and healthy snack.
26. Smoothies: Whip up some goodness into a drinkable snack!
27. Pears: So sweet and juicy
28. Raisins: Everyone loves these little guys!
29. Dark chocolate: A couple of nibbles of dark chocolate can satisfy the sweet tooth while providing lots of antioxidants
30. Pineapple: On its own or as part of a fruit salad, sliced pineapple is heavenly
31. Mango: Speaking of heavenly, mango has got to be one of the most delicious foods on the planet
32. Sweet peas: Definitely a Part-Time Paleo snack
33. Homemade fruit roll-ups: Puree some fruit, pour a thin layer on a parchment-lined baking sheet, and bake it at your oven's lowest temperature for 6–8 hours. Or use a food dehydrator if you have one.

SNACK AND TREAT RECIPES

Trail Mix

Yields 3 cups

 1 cup raw pumpkin seeds
 ½ cup chopped almonds
 ⅓ cup pistachios
 ⅓ cup pecans
 1 tablespoon coconut oil, melted
 1 ½ tablespoons maple syrup
 1 teaspoon cinnamon
 ¼ teaspoon ground nutmeg
 ¼ teaspoon sea salt
 ⅓ cup chopped dried dates
 ½ cup unsweetened shredded coconut

Preheat oven to 375 degrees. On a parchment-lined sheet pan, toss together all ingredients except dates and coconut. Roast in the oven for 7–10 minutes, or until the mixture is slightly toasted and fragrant. Remove from the oven and toss in the dates and coconut. Let cool completely and store in an airtight container.

Chocolate Coconut Cookie Balls

Yields 1 dozen small cookie balls

 8 large Medjool dates, pitted
 1 ½ cups raw almonds
 2 tablespoons coconut butter
 4 tablespoons mini dark chocolate chips
 1 pinch sea salt
 ½ cup unsweetened shredded coconut

In a food processor, pulse together dates, almonds, and coconut butter. Once the mix is smooth, add chocolate and salt, and pulse two more times. With a spoon, scoop out some of the mixture and roll into balls. Roll the balls in the coconut and store in an airtight container in the refrigerator until ready to serve.

Ants on a Boat

Yields 4 servings

    4 tablespoons almond butter
    2 medium Honeycrisp apples, halved and cored
    2 tablespoons raw honey
    20 plump raisins

Spread 1 tablespoon of almond butter on each apple half. Drizzle honey over each. Place 5 raisins in a row on each apple half. Serve right away.

Turkey Roll-Ups

Yields 4 servings

    8 slices nitrate-free, organic turkey breast
    1 medium cucumber, peeled and sliced into thin strips
    ¼ cup Paleo-friendly guacamole
    2 roma tomatoes, sliced thin

On a clean work surface, lay out all the turkey slices. In the center of each slice of turkey, place a couple of cucumber strips. Spread an even layer of guacamole over cucumbers and top with a couple of tomatoes. Roll turkey with all the fixings into a tight spiral and serve.

Serving suggestion: Dip the turkey roll-ups in some yummy hummus!

Chocolaty Frozen Berry Pops

Yields 4 servings

4 wooden skewers
1 pint strawberries, washed and hulled
1 pint dark sweet cherries, pitted
1 banana, sliced
2 cups dark chocolate chips, melted

On each wooden skewer, slide strawberries, cherries, and banana slices, alternating until each skewer is full. Dip the skewers in the melted chocolate until evenly coated on all sides. Place the dipped skewers in an airtight container so that none of them are touching. Place in the freezer for at least 2 hours before serving.

Dr. Wahls's Kale Chips

Makes a big bowlful

6–8 cups chopped fresh kale, hard stems removed
2 tablespoons olive oil or melted coconut oil
1 tablespoon apple cider vinegar or fresh lemon juice
½ teaspoon sea salt

Place a rack on the lowest shelf in your oven. Preheat to 350 degrees.

In a large mixing bowl, add the chopped kale, and drizzle with oil and apple cider vinegar. Massage the oil and vinegar into the kale with your hands to penetrate the kale, for up to 5 minutes or until the kale starts to smell like freshly cut grass. Spread the massaged kale on a cookie sheet.

Place sheet on lowest rack of oven and bake for 10 minutes.

Remove from oven and stir so that kale can get crispy all over. Bake for another 8–12 minutes, or until kale is crispy. It should be just lightly browned and crispy to the touch. If kale still bends rather than crackles when you touch it, it isn't done yet—return it to the oven and watch it constantly so it won't burn! Turn down the heat if it is getting too brown.

When it's done, remove kale from the oven and sprinkle with sea salt.

Paleo Granola Bars

Makes 16 to 20

1 cup pumpkin seeds

1 cup sunflower seeds

1 cup slivered almonds

½ cup almond meal

1 cup unsweetened dried cranberries

1 cup unsweetened dried coconut

½ cup almond butter

½ cup raw honey

1 teaspoon vanilla extract

¼–½ teaspoon sea salt (or to taste)

¼ teaspoon nutmeg

½ teaspoon cinnamon

Place a piece of parchment paper into the bottom of a 9 × 13 baking dish.

In a large mixing bowl, add first six ingredients and mix well.

In a medium saucepan, add remaining ingredients and cook over medium heat. Once mixture is bubbling, pour over the top of the nut mixture and quickly stir to incorporate.

Pour warm mixture into the baking dish, using clean hands to press flat. Allow to sit until hardened, about an hour or so. (Note: On hot and/or humid days, it won't harden well on its own; a freezer will do wonders once the mixture has cooled.)

Cut into bars (they will still be a little crumbly), and serve!

PART-TIME PALEO TREATS

The key to living a Part-Time Paleo lifestyle is getting in as much nutrition as you can through quality food. This means we don't fill up on empty calories and processed foods.

But, that being said, we don't deprive ourselves of treats *all* the time. They're just different treats!

You can find recipes for Paleo brownies and cookies to satisfy your sweet tooth at PartTimePaleoBook.com. These recipes use natural sweeteners and gluten-free flours so you can splurge without putting garbage in your body.

A FINAL WORD FROM LEANNE

The Part-Time Paleo lifestyle is not a fad. This way of eating and living has healed my body and helped keep my weight under control, and it has me feeling better than I've ever felt in my life.

I will not go back to eating the way I once did, not because I'm not allowed to eat grains or sugar, but because I don't want to feel that way again. I am done with feeling bloated and lethargic after bingeing on freshly baked bread. I don't want to be chained to sugar for the rest of my life.

I have taken control of my health and, let me tell you, it feels amazing.

A few years ago, I wrote a book with the Fly Lady, Marla Cilley, called *Body Clutter: Love Your Body, Love Yourself.* In that book, we talked about getting rid of the emotional crap and the lifestyle crap that causes the body clutter to cling to your butt and thighs.

Following a Part-Time Paleo lifestyle has helped me to truly embrace the concepts we wrote about in that book.

I am worth a good night's rest. I am worth the massages, the smoothies, and the trips to the gym.

Following the principles of the Paleo lifestyle makes it simple to stay healthy because it naturally forces you to eliminate the foods that pack weight on and make you unhealthy. This *Part-Time Paleo* book can be considered a kind of extension of that book Marla and I wrote together. If you've read *Body Clutter,* you know how to get rid of the negative thinking that packs on pounds. And when you go Part-Time Paleo, you'll know once and for all how to maintain a healthy weight.

Body Clutter taught us that it's okay to not be perfect. *Part-Time Paleo*—by its very nature—is also about not being perfect! It's about taking the principles of a healthy lifestyle and doing the best that you can with applying them. Let's face facts. How many times have you started a diet, a plan, a "lifestyle" . . . only to pitch it as far as you could throw it because you couldn't do it "perfectly"? I get that, and I also get that Paleo perfectionists out there are dying to make you feel guilty because you like some Parmesan on top of that delicious Paleo minestrone.

Relax!

You can have your cheese (if you follow the rules) and eat it, too!

RESOURCES

Throughout this book I've referenced some of my favorite resources for living a Part-Time Paleo life.

Here is more information about those resources and where you can find them:

All-in-One Smoothie Mix. An avid smoothie drinker, I was so unhappy with the different types of protein powders on the market that I decided to go ahead and create something myself that I could use in my daily blender specials! Saving Dinner All-in-One Smoothie Mixes are made with chlorella and pea and potato protein, which are all types of low-allergenicity proteins. These mixes are free of soy, egg, peanuts, dairy, and gluten, and they contain no artificial ingredients or fructose. All-in-One Smoothie Mixes are available in chocolate, vanilla, and chai flavors. Find more at SavingDinner.com.

Bulletproof Coffee.* Bulletproof Coffee is a staple in my house. This coffee makes you feel fabulous! The beans are meant to be enjoyed black or to make Bulletproof Coffee, which is made by blending black coffee with organic grass-fed butter for a delicious, creamy drink. Get your beans (and more information) at BulletproofExec.com.

Coconut Aminos. Because of the health concerns surrounding genetically modified soy, I avoid soy sauce and I suggest that you avoid it, too. There's a great alternative on the market called coconut aminos. Made from sea salt and the sap from coconut palms, it's packed with minerals and vitamins and tastes and looks just like the soy sauce you're familiar with. It can be difficult to find coconut aminos, depending on where you live, but you can find it online at CoconutSecret.com.

FiberMender. Saving Dinner FiberMender is my own creation, and I use it in my smoothies every day to help keep me regular and to keep my GI flora nice and balanced. Find out more at SavingDinner.com.

Green PolkaDot Box. This resource wasn't mentioned in the book, but if you don't have a good health food store nearby, the Green PolkaDot Box may just be your saving grace. Like Costco for health nuts, Green PolkaDot Box is a Web store that sells all those health foods you can't find in regular stores. It works on a club membership model, and the price of membership includes many perks. Find out more at GreenPolka DotBox.com.

Gut and Psychology Syndrome **(GAPS) Book.** Dr. Natasha Campbell-McBride believes there is a link between learning disabilities, our food and drink, and the condition of our digestive system. *Gut and Psychology Syndrome* is about food as a natural treatment for ADD, ADHD, autism, depression, dyslexia, dyspraxia, and schizophrenia. Find out more at GutAndPsychologySyndrome.com.

---

* My friend David Asprey, aka the Bulletproof Executive, worked tirelessly to find the best coffee beans on the planet.

Terry Wahls. As I mentioned at the beginning of this book, Dr. Terry Wahls forever changed the way I look at nutrition. This inspirational woman beat progressive multiple sclerosis by implementing the principles of the Paleo diet in her life. Find out more about her at TerryWahls.com.

The Wizard's Organic Saucery. I buy all of my hot sauce and my Worcestershire sauce from the Wizard's line of organic sauces. There's a gluten-free option and even a vegan option. Order at EdwardAndSons .com.

Get access to all sorts of additional information and resources that will help you on your Part-Time Paleo journey and beyond at PartTime PaleoBook.com

RESEARCH

Cordain, Loren. *The Paleo Answer: 7 Days to Lose Weight, Feel Great, Stay Young.* Hoboken, NJ: John Wiley & Sons, 2012.

Konner, Melvin. "Eat Like a Hunter-Gatherer." The Official Website of Melvin Konner, MD, PhD. http://www.melvinkonner.com/index.php?option=com_wordpress&p=17&Itemid=72.

Lindeberg, Staffan. "Our Research." http://www.staffanlindeberg.com/OurResearch.html.

Taubes, Gary. *Why We Get Fat: And What to Do About It.* New York: Alfred A. Knopf, 2010.

INDEX